Don't Quit, Get Fit

I have known Vicki for more than 15 years as we have worked together in the health and fitness industry, and I have always been impressed with her personal commitment to fitness, her honesty about her challenges, and her perseverance to overcome any obstacles in her path. This book is packed with practical thoughts and action points that can help you overcome your personal obstacles as you choose fitness and health. It is a life-changing book. Don't miss it!

Jeannie Blocher
President of Body & Soul Fitness

Vicki Heath cares for people! Her vibrant spirit will cheer you on to be your best, and each word in this book will help extend your life and bring you more joy, hope and enthusiasm. I know, because she is one of the cheerleaders in my life who has helped me live longer and stronger!

Pam Farrel
Author of more than 34 Books, including the bestselling *Men Are Like Waffles, Women Are Like Spaghetti; 10 Secrets to Living Smart, Strong and Savvy* and *10 Best Decisions a Woman Can Make*

Don't Quit, Get Fit will show you how to honor God with your body. Vicki reveals in an open and transparent way her own struggles with staying fit and what she does about it. What I like most about this book is that she provides specific solutions to specific excuses for an unhealthy lifestyle. This book is packed with helpful tips that can change your life forever.

Steve Reynolds
Author of *Bod4God* and founder of Losing to Live

Don't Quit, Get Fit is a practical, attention-grabbing fitness book that—along with giving plans for success—addresses all our excuses for not getting fit. This book teaches how to get spiritually, mentally, emotionally and physically fit for a lifetime. Yes, that is possible!

Lauraine Snelling
Bestselling fiction author of 70-plus novels, including *Valley of Dreams* and *On Hummingbird Wings*

Don't Quit
GET FIT

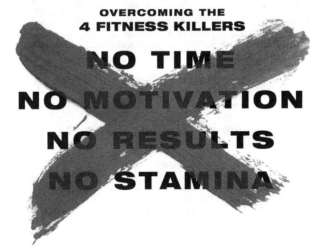

**OVERCOMING THE
4 FITNESS KILLERS**

NO TIME
NO MOTIVATION
NO RESULTS
NO STAMINA

VICKI HEATH

Regal

From Gospel Light
Ventura, California, U.S.A.

Published by Regal
From Gospel Light
Ventura, California, U.S.A.
www.regalbooks.com
Printed in the U.S.A.

Library of Congress Cataloging-in-Publication Data
Heath, Vicki.
Don't quit, get fit : overcoming the 4 fitness killers (no time, no motivation, no results,
no stamina) / Vicki Heath.
p. cm.
Includes bibliographical references (p.   ).
ISBN 978-0-8307-5950-7 (hard cover)
1. Physical fitness. 2. Physical fitness—Religious aspects—Christianity. I. Title.
RA781.H3775 2011
613.7—dc23
2011027567

Contents

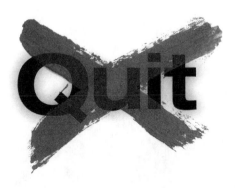

FOREWORD

I met Vicki Heath when her youngest son, McKenzie, was a baby. Mac is now in college, but it seems like just yesterday when we met. Vicki excels as a wife and mother, and she and her husband, Rob, live in beautiful Edisto Beach, South Carolina, where Rob is pastor of Edisto Beach Baptist Church. Vicki has pursued wellness for almost 20 years, and she and Rob have raised their four children to be vibrantly healthy adults in every area—spiritually, mentally, emotionally and physically.

Vicki is a motivating leader of both First Place 4 Health and Body & Soul Fitness classes, and her members adore her. I have picked up so many great tips from Vicki. One of my favorites is to keep my workout shoes in my car so I can walk when I have to wait somewhere. This has been a valuable tip, because we all spend a lot of time waiting.

In *Don't Quit, Get Fit*, Vicki shares how she learned to pursue a life of fitness and how her love of exercise has spilled over into every area of her life. As you read this book, you will be motivated and inspired to begin or continue your own journey to a healthy and fit life. You will discover your sustaining motivation so that you will never give up and never give out.

I love and admire Vicki Heath, and all of us at First Place 4 Health and Body & Soul Fitness are more than a little proud of Vicki. I know you will love her as much as we do after you read this book.

Carole Lewis
First Place 4 Health National Director

1

Hope 4 Me?

Has there ever been a time in your life when you simply couldn't get it together and improve your health? Have you ever found yourself daydreaming about how great life would be if you could just get in shape?

Until the fall of 1993, I had been able to stay in pretty good shape. Not perfect, but good enough. But in 1993 I became completely stuck. I would tell myself I already knew how to get in shape, and I would daydream about what my life would look like when I did. But if you don't move, you don't lose—and I wasn't moving. I needed help, but I was too proud to ask, so I just kept daydreaming.

On one particular day that Fall, three significant situations converged that helped me begin an amazing journey.

First, my fourth child was almost one year old. While this child was a very pleasant surprise, he was still a surprise! I managed my eating and exercise pretty well at first, but eventually it was all I could do to get out of bed and care for my four children, much less exercise. That led to the second significant situation: I gained quite a bit of weight. Soon I weighed more then I had ever weighed in my entire life. I could no longer pretend to not care. I *had* to deal with the issue of weight and how to lose it. After my previous pregnancies, I had managed to eventually lose the extra pounds, but this time was different. I don't know if it was my age or just a lack of time and motivation. Around that time, we bought our first Internet-ready computer, which was the third significant situation.

Sitting at our new computer, I experienced a life-changing crisis. As I booted up the computer for the first time, it asked me to create a password. I needed something I would not forget, something that I thought about every day. The perfect password came way too quickly: I thought about my weight every day. Discouraged and feeling hopeless about the size of my body, I was becoming convinced that I would never lose the weight. Needless to say, I was at a turning point in my life. As I sat at my computer, the password came to me in the form of a prayer: "Lord, is there any hope for me to lose this weight? Can You help me? Can You help me help myself?" I knew in my mind all the things I needed to do to lose the weight, but the feeling of hopelessness was overwhelming—and thus came the password "hope4me." In effect, this password became my daily prayer: "Lord, is there any hope for me?"

About the same time, my dear sweet mother-in-law, Lou Heath, saw my struggle and mentioned a new weight-loss group called First Place 4 Health, which was meeting at her church in Nashville. "It's like Weight Watchers for Christians," she told me by way of encouragement. First Place 4 Health was having a training meeting in Ocala, Florida, and a glimmer of hope was born in my heart.

I called Melanie, a dear friend who knew and understood my struggle, to ask if she was interested in taking a road trip with me to learn about this new Christian way of weight loss. Since she was struggling with this same issue, she of course was interested. When we arrived at the meeting, I immediately noticed that the other hundred or so attendees seemed to be in the same shape I was. I was immediately encouraged. Several testimonies were shared on how First Place 4 Health had been a godsend in their lives, and then the attendees dispersed to various classrooms to get started on the program. When I entered a classroom and climbed on the scale, I said to myself, *I never have to weigh this much again.* It's now 17 years later, and I haven't!

After arriving back home, my friend and I enlisted a small group of women who shared our weight problems and frustrations. I made them swear an oath that we would tell no one what we were doing, in case of failure. What little faith I had! Failure had become an old familiar friend, and I did not want to renew that relationship yet again. Our group met in secret on Sunday nights and, despite my lack of faith, we all experienced success.

That was almost two decades ago, and what a journey it has been. I have learned at the feet of the Lord of His plan for my life and how to walk in His way, committed to a lifetime of wellness. Over the years, my quiet time with the Lord has always encouraged me to persevere, even when I feel like quitting. When I pursue God, He blesses me with wisdom, knowledge and an understanding of the truth that keeps me on the road to wellness. He has led me to encourage others to press on with perseverance toward their goals. I can't wait to share with you all that He has shown me. Much of it I have learned the hard way, but I *have* learned, and so can you.

Of all the verses of Scripture that have impacted my life, Hebrews 12:1-3 has served as a flagship of hope. In these verses I have found my wellness theology!

> Therefore, since we are surrounded by such a great cloud of witnesses, let us throw off everything that hinders and the sin that so easily entangles, and let us run with perseverance the race marked out for us. Let us fix our eyes on Jesus, the author and perfecter of our faith, who for the joy set before him endured the cross, scorning its shame, and sat down at the right hand of the throne of God. Consider him who endured such opposition from sinful men, so that you will not grow weary and lose heart.

From these three verses, God has taught me a ton about not giving up—what I call my running theology.

When I started on my journey, I had so much to overcome. I had never been a disciplined person, and I realized early on that getting healthy and losing weight was going to cost me something. It was going to require some of the hardest work I had ever done. The same will be true for you. It will cost you some of your money, your time, your energy, and you will have to do without the things you like to eat that are not good for you. A life based on the principles of First Place 4 Health is a life of *discipline* and *sacrifice*—two words that are countercultural today.

Of course, the fruits of discipline and sacrifice have been so empowering and rewarding for me that I am committed for life! I hope you will experience the same joy and commitment. Let's walk together through these three verses and learn what God can teach us about this race we call life.

Lesson #1: Run Free

Hebrews 12:1 tells us to "throw off everything that hinders and entangles" us. God wants us to run the race of life without being burdened. These words paint a picture of a runner carrying items that would prevent him or her from running quickly. Every runner needs to get rid of excess baggage. I had two areas in my life that were weighing me down as I began the race toward wellness: laziness and dishonesty. I hated to admit it at first, but I was lazy! I did not want to do the hard work; I wanted God to do the hard work. After all, He is totally capable of making me fat free. I was ready for Him to perform a weight-loss miracle. When I felt especially disgusted with myself, I would pray my fat prayer:

> *Dear Lord, I know You can take the fat away. Please, God, let me wake up in the morning and have it gone. I will praise Your name forever. Many people will come into the Kingdom as a result of this miracle.*

I simply did not want to do the hard work of keeping track of my food and exercising. I did not want to be obedient and sacrifice anything. My laziness also reared its ugly head every morning when the alarm went off. I did not want to wake up early to spend time with God. Getting up early for a quiet time with God takes work and preparation. I despised my laziness and in my heart I wanted to be close with God and to pursue His wholeness, but in my body I pursued laziness. Laziness had entangled me, and I wanted out of the knot.

How did things begin to change? The first thing I did was ask God to forgive me for my lazy attitude and actions. Being honest about past laziness, I repented and decided to change. I had to make a plan to change my thinking and then to change my behavior. Throwing off the laziness that so easily entangled me and hindered me from my pursuit of God, I had to next confront my dishonesty. For many years, I had lied to myself about the importance of controlling my weight. I would tell myself that it really did not matter. God looked on the inside of a person, not the outside, right? True, but God also gave us our lives and the responsibility to live as fully and completely as possible. As a pastor's wife and mother of four children, I knew deep down that God wanted me to be healthy, so I could live out His purpose for those in my care. My dishonesty kept me from confronting the deeper issue in my life: guilt. For some of us, the first weight we need to lose is the weight we carry on our shoulders: the guilt and shame from past failures. Once I began to be honest with God about who I was and my failures in the past, I began to feel the freedom to run light, unburdened by guilt.

But dishonesty continued to hinder my walk with the Lord and my wellness journey. Throwing it off was hard, and keeping it off was even harder! I knew that I needed help to stick with it. Since I had a tendency toward being dishonest about my weight, I needed someone else to weigh me every week, so I found someone else to keep my numbers honest. God requires truth in our inmost parts.

Just as God has helped me, so too He wants to help you throw off the things that are keeping you from running light. What is slowing you down? Take time now to ask the Holy Spirit to show you the areas in your life that you need to confront. Allow God to speak to your heart and give you direction. As you discover what's holding you back, throw it off, so you can run light and experience freedom.

Lesson #2: Run Steady

The second valuable running lesson I gained from Hebrews 12:1-3 was to "run with perseverance." The best runners in the world pace themselves. They run to complete the entire race. Their goal is not to just have a good beginning but to also run well the entire race. If you run steadily and consistently, you'll finish the race and meet your goal.

We live in a culture of instant gratification. We do not gain weight and get out of shape in just a few weeks or months. Why in the world do we think we can lose weight and get fit in just a couple of months? I strongly encourage you to give God a year of your very best efforts; then you will achieve success. You will encounter many obstacles on your journey to get fit, but whenever you do, buckle down and persevere.

Obstacles in Your Path

What is an obstacle? An obstacle is anything that stands in the way or opposes you. A military obstacle training course is filled with things to overcome or negotiate, such as hurdles, fences, walls and ditches. Wellness obstacles might be losing a job, having to care for an aging parent, or grieving the loss of a loved one. An obstacle could also be a person, such as your spouse or a close friend, who for whatever reason does not want you to succeed. Many times obstacles come in the form of injuries or are personal habits that seem impossible to overcome. Things *will* happen, and things *will* get in the way. But when you have the right perspective, you will be able to succeed.

First, remember that obstacles are to be expected. Jesus clearly said that we would have things in our lives that would make it difficult to walk closely with God and pursue His plan for our lives. He promised that if we follow Him, we would have a boatload of difficulties. In John 16:33 Jesus said, "In this world you will have trouble. But take heart! I have overcome the world." So when you decide to follow God's best for your life—when you put God first—you'll have troubles. The great news is that Jesus promises He will be with you every step of the way. So when you confront an obstacle, there is no need to be discouraged: God knew it was coming. Stop complaining about the obstacle and start figuring out your next move.

Talking about the trouble he faced, Paul wrote in a letter to a young leader named Timothy:

> You ... know all about my ... persecutions and sufferings—what kinds of things happened to me in Antioch, Iconium and Lystra, the persecutions I endured. Yet the Lord rescued me from all of them. In fact, everyone who wants to live a godly life in Christ Jesus will be persecuted (2 Tim. 3:10-12).

Paul wanted to encourage Timothy to not give up when obstacles appeared in his path. Paul faced the real possibility of being arrested, being beaten and even dying for his faith. These things won't confront most of us, but we will still face obstacles that will hamper us from keeping God first in our lives.

Dealing with Obstacles

There are several approaches we can take when faced by an obstacle. One approach is to quit, turn around and go back to the way we were. Paralyzed with fear, anger and bitterness, we are tempted to simply give up. The book of Hebrews was written to a community facing the obstacle of persecution, and some new Christians were tempted to go back to their old ways of living. When the writer says "run with perseverance," we learn that giving up is not an option that God offers. What else can we do? Let me suggest two options that have worked in my life.

The first option is to slow down, catch your breath and jump over the obstacle! It takes faith to jump. It's scary. Every time I take a leap of faith, I am nervous and my knees shake. But that's okay. We need to be humble and go ahead and jump. When we follow Jesus, our first step is to get down on our knees. When we admit our inability to do things on our own—when we slow down and cry out to God for help—then God will literally lift us over the obstacle in front of us. James 4:10 says, "Humble yourselves before the Lord, and *he will lift you up*" (emphasis added)! Once you've positioned yourself to jump and you know that God is with you, take the next step and leap right over that obstacle.

Donna faced her obstacle, a weight of 189 pounds, by adding exercise to her routine. Listen to her story in her own words:

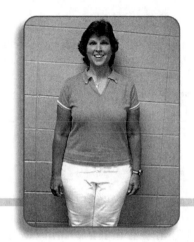 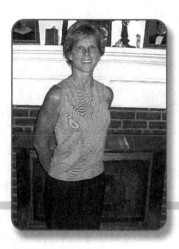

DONNA CONERLY

In January 2009, I started getting serious about my weight problem and joined a First Place 4 Health class in Brandon, Mississippi. I realized that exercise needed to be a big part of my success, so I started walking shortly after beginning the program. I started slowly, walking alone at my own pace. I know that walking consistently five days a week really helped my weight loss.

By August 2009, I had found a few First Place 4 Health buddies to hold me accountable, and they asked me to join them on their regular Saturday walk/run. I swallowed my pride and gave it a shot. That first Saturday I was exhausted, but I was determined to try to keep up with them. Even though I spent the whole hour looking at the rear ends of my friends who stayed ahead of me, I did not quit. As the weeks rolled by, I became stronger and faster, and I began to see even more weight loss. I was so encouraged that I began to change my solo workouts by adding some trotting. I would walk a short distance and then trot the same short distance. As I consistently did this day after day, I could gradually trot longer distances. Today I have lost a total of 61 pounds. My starting weight was 189, and this morning my weight was 128. Thank You, Lord Jesus! For only through Him have I been able to reach my current level of fitness. Today I am stronger and more fit than I have ever been in my 52 years of life.

I completed my fourth half-marathon on April 30, 2011, with my fastest time ever of 2 hours 2 minutes. I completed my first full marathon in October 2010, finishing in 5 hours and 50 minutes. And I plan to run my next full marathon on October 15, 2011. I hope to run it in 5 hours or less. On average I now run 20 to 25 miles every week. About a year ago, I incorporated weight training in my exercise routine, lifting free weights at home several days a week. I love the running and exercise that are part of my daily life now. I no longer dread or hate it. I spent so many years not caring for my body, the temple of the Holy Spirit. But thanks be to God for His mercy and grace, today my body is a strong, fit and healthy temple in which He dwells!

All for Him.

Remember what Jesus said: "I have overcome the world." Together, you and Jesus can overcome the obstacles that get in your way. Remember what Paul said about the trials that he went through: "The Lord rescued me from all of them." The psalmist says it like this: "I cried out to God for help; I cried out to God to hear me. When I was in distress, I sought the Lord" (Ps. 77:1-2). If you want to run steady, you need to pray steady and then jump over the obstacle.

The second option is to walk through the obstacle. Sometimes an obstacle may come in the form of something you may not be able to jump over. It may be something for which God does not give a quick fix, but rather leads you through the longer process of healing and hope. During such times, you need to fully depend on God, even when it seems you have no place to set your feet. Psalm 69:1-2 often carries me through when I encounter these obstacles:

Save me, O God, for the waters have come up to my neck,
I sink in the miry depth where there is no foothold.

Psalm 40:1-3 says it this way:

I waited patiently for the LORD; he turned to me and heard my cry. He lifted me out of the slimy pit, out of the mud and mire; he set my feet on a rock and gave me a firm place to stand. He put a new song in my mouth, a hymn of praise to our God. Many will see and fear and put their trust in the LORD.

We will all face times when we simply need to persevere through a difficulty. When there is no easy way to jump over an obstacle, we just need to work our way through it. Giving up is not an option. We persevere so that we will find the success that God intends for our lives.

A man met a guru in the road and asked him, "Which way is success?" The bearded sage did not speak but pointed to a place off in the distance. Thrilled by the prospect of quick and easy success, the man rushed off in the appropriate direction. Suddenly, there was a loud splat. Eventually, the man limped back, tattered and stunned, assuming he must have misinterpreted the message. He repeated his question to the guru, who again pointed silently in the same direction. Once again the man obediently walked off. This time the splat was deafening; and when the man crawled back, he was bloody, broken, tattered and irate. "I asked you which way is success!" he screamed at the guru. "I followed the direction you indicated! And all I got was splatted! No more of this pointing! Talk!" Only then did the guru speak, and what he said was this: "Success *is* that way. Just a little past splat."

When we run steady and persevere, we make it beyond the splat!

Lesson #3: Never Run Alone

I can tell you right now, there will be days when you will need help from others. We are not designed to live life by ourselves. Our passage from Hebrews begins by describing how we are surrounded by a "great cloud of witnesses." Imagine being in a football stadium with everyone in the stands there to cheer us on. We were not meant to do this alone. God made us to encourage one another. We can find encouragement from witnesses who've already succeeded in their walk toward wholeness and from those seeking to walk closely with God today.

Ecclesiastes 4:9-10 says, "Two are better than one, because they have a good return for their work: If one falls down, his friend can help him up." Remember when you were a kid and you were outside playing with friends and you came to a wall or fence you could not climb over? What did you do? You figured out how to help each other over. My sister Val and I grew up on military bases all over the United States, and because we were so good at clasping fingers together to make a step for the other, there was no fence we could not climb, no place we could not reach. We counted on each other for help.

There will be times when you are confronted by obstacles so seemingly insurmountable that you cannot get over them by yourself. If you try to go it alone, you may end up a bloody, broken mess. There is nothing like a friend with whom you can be honest and know that he or she has your back and will be there for you. We all need people around us who can lift us up, carry us over and walk us through the hard times in our lives.

"Carry each other's burdens, and in this way you will fulfill the law of Christ" (Gal. 6:2). You must create a personal support system around yourself. Enlist one or two faithful friends with whom you can be gut-level honest, who will be there for you when you are tempted to quit or give in to temptation. The Church provides the perfect place for this kind of support. If you are not connected to a local body of believers, consider taking that step.

Remember that you are not the first to follow God's plan, and you won't be the last. As you study the Bible, you will find that "a great cloud of witnesses" is there to encourage and support you through difficult times.

Lesson #4: Run Your Own Race

One of the worst mistakes novice runners make during a big race is to watch more experienced runners and try to run their race. Instead of sticking to the plan laid out by their coach, they follow the crowd. The book of Hebrews warns against that by telling us to "run with perseverance the *race marked out for [us]*." God did not design each of us to be the same; instead, we are designed to fit together like a puzzle, like parts of one body, working together to perform a given task.

One of the hardest things I deal with is comparing myself to others. As a fitness instructor, I find that the comparisons can be brutal. I work in an industry that expects you to have a perfect body and to stay ahead of the aging process. The reality is that I do not have a perfect body and that I am getting older every day! It is dangerous for me to compare myself to people in their twenties. My race also involves overcoming that laziness I mentioned earlier. I work around the laziness by placing myself in a teaching role. Instead of trying to do it for myself, I become the teacher who is responsible for others. In this way, I've been able to overcome what I wouldn't do for myself.

God has a race marked out specifically for you, so don't be tempted to compare yourself with those around you. There is a race you were designed for from the beginning of the world. You are gifted in so many ways that are different from everyone else.

There is no one else exactly like you! You are an individual who was uniquely created. I love how the psalmist describes this in Psalm 139:

> You [God] created my inmost being; you knit me together in my mother's womb. I praise you because I am fearfully and wonderfully made; your works are wonderful, I know that full well. My frame was not hidden from you when I was made in the secret place. When I was woven together in the depths of the earth, your eyes saw my unformed body. All the days ordained for me were written in your book before one of them came to be (vv. 13-16).

Run the way God designed you to run. Learn to understand your strengths and weaknesses. Operate within your strengths and around your weaknesses.

Nothing about you is a mistake. God made you with those arms, those legs and those ears, so stop comparing yourself to others! Learn to appreciate your uniqueness and develop an attitude of gratitude for who you are. You've got your own race to run.

Lesson #5: Run Focused

There will be plenty of things along the way to distract you from your wellness goals. You will be tempted to stop putting God first in the midst of your busy life. You will be tempted to look to something new that promises "Lose 30 pounds in two weeks!" or "Lose weight without exercising!" Do not be fooled. Fixing your eyes on Jesus, "the author and perfecter" of your faith, is the secret to your success (Heb. 12:2).

The life of faith and wellness is fraught with the temptation to take the easy way out. Jesus faced a similar temptation when He began His journey on earth. Satan tempted Him by saying that he would give Jesus all the authority in the earth if only Jesus would turn and worship him (see Luke 4:6). Jesus knew that the way to long-term, life-giving success was God's plan of obedience and not the easy way by accepting the deceiver's gift, so Jesus responded, "Worship the Lord your God and serve him only" (Luke 4:8).

As you will discover, wellness is not simply about losing weight. Wellness is about living the life that God intends for you. Taking the easy way out will not help you receive everything God has for you.

Jesus began this good work in you, and He will complete it. He is at work all the time to help you stay focused. Look to Jesus for everything in your life. All you need for godliness is in the relationship you develop with Christ Himself. Run to Him and look to Him for strength, for power, for grace, for forgiveness, for a new day and for hope.

You will discover the same password for the race called life that I discovered: There is hope for you!

2

Lies that Steal, Kill and Destroy

Abby was frustrated, depressed *and* hopeful.

She was frustrated because she had allowed her weight to get out of control, she was depressed because her heart broke whenever she thought about her weight, and she was hopeful because she had come to live with her aunt, who was committed to doing whatever it took to get her back on the path to wellness.

When my niece, Abby, came to live with us for three months, she was cautiously optimistic that things would change. Little did we know just how defeated Abby really felt. We had to start somewhere, so on that first day I explained to her how it was going to work: Every day we would read our Bible, exercise and eat quality foods in proper quantities, and once a week we would weigh in.

Just the mention of getting on the scale caused Abby to go pale. The first time she stepped on the scale, I could see her fear and trepidation. The numbers shot up, and Abby fell down. She began to cry, saying, "I am such a loser. I will never be able to do this. I have so much to lose!"

I realized at that moment that her weight was not the real problem: Abby was allowing the scale to define her. She believed that the scale measured how valuable she was. The scale does *not* do that. Abby was a beautiful, smart and lovely girl who had allowed a number on a scale to make her feel worthless.

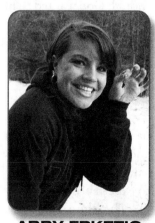

ABBY FRKETIC

I told her, "Never again will the scale define you. You are defined by Christ, and He finds you perfect." Abby's first step was to begin to see herself as God sees her. It's your first step as well.

How Jesus Confronted the Lies

Do you know what got Jesus fired up? Jesus seized opportunities to confront lies that prevented people from becoming who they were meant to be. One day, Jesus and His disciples came across a man who had been blind from birth. The disciples asked a reasonable question (for their culture and time period): Was it the man's sin or that of his parents that caused him to be born blind? The Jewish leaders believed and taught that such birth defects were punishment for sin: Either the baby had sinned in the womb or the parents had sinned. Case closed. But Jesus did not hold with this belief.

Jesus' answer still echoes today: "Neither this man nor his parents sinned . . . but this happened so that the work of God might be displayed in his life" (John 9:3). Jesus began to break down the lies and bring life.

To make a long story short, Jesus healed the man on the Sabbath and put the religious leaders in an uproar. At the end of a long confrontation, in which the man acknowledged that Jesus came from God, the Pharisees shouted a lie to bring the man down, even though God wanted to lift him up: "You were steeped in sin at birth; how dare you lecture us!" (John 9:34). They wanted this man to believe that he would never be anything more than a blind sinner who did not deserve God's grace. Jesus confronted that lie that wanted to steal away the man's life. He wants to confront our lies as well.

A little later on, Jesus told the crowds, "The thief comes only to steal and kill and destroy; I have come that they may have life, and have it to the full" (John 10:10). Jesus is the same yesterday, today and forever, and the thieves are still trying to steal our joy, deny our value and destroy our ability to experience life as God intends for us to experience it.

The blind man moved from darkness to light because He listened to the voice that told him he was more than just a blind man—

he was a child loved by God who could be used to bring God glory. You, too, will begin to move toward wellness when you allow God's words of love to speak deeply and richly into your life and as you confront the lies that attempt to steal your joy, kill your desire to get healthy and destroy any possibility of living the full and abundant life that God has for you.

Read about how Judi confronted the lies about eating that existed in her life:

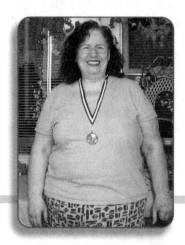

JUDI LEE GRANT

How can I begin to express all that God has done these past 12 weeks, as He lovingly pursued me and I responded with the mustard seed of faith He gave me?

The Lord has helped me to take control of my physical actions: eating correct portions (by putting individual servings in snack bags), accepting that it is okay to feel hunger pangs and tracking food daily online.

I've also come to realize that my desire to overeat has less to do with certain triggers (feeling like I cannot control myself) and more to do with sin. My flesh wants to overeat and I've been giving in instead of seeking God. In Christ I have found true freedom to enjoy all that God has for me.

Yes, I have to have personal responsibility and accountability. No, I don't want to be tempted, so I need to make wise choices about what I expose myself to. However, I am no longer afraid of specific foods. They are not what caused my weight problem. I don't need to be afraid of foods at a party, church supper or holiday meal. Those special foods will always be around.

I have to access controls inside of me through the Holy Spirit. Yes, I choose to have healthy choices (nutrient-dense foods and snacks) in my house; however, I no longer fear that a particular food will destroy my control. I really have Jesus Christ, God the Father and the Holy Spirit living in me. The power that raised Jesus Christ from the dead is available to help me with food and exercise issues.

I no longer buy into the lie that I have no power over my overeating and exercise. The words of Satan (the father of lies) no longer control my emotional response. I trust the words of my Savior who gives me the ability to move forward and control physical and emotional cravings for certain foods.

I am no longer a slave to sin but a servant of righteousness. I focus on God, not my next meal or snack. Food can be a blessing to us, not a curse. Food is for nourishment and fellowship with others.

As a result of this truth, I've made a myriad of changes in my life. I can live this new lifestyle through Christ who strengthens me. I am more cognizant of my positive and negative emotions that used to impact my eating choices. I am aware of what foods I choose and more knowledgeable about their benefits. I memorize Scripture and allow God's words to fill my thoughts. My attitude toward exercise has changed, and now I look forward to moving more and finding new trails to walk on. I am getting out more whatever the weather may be. I am less sedentary, watch less television and go to bed earlier. I met or exceeded my weight and measurement goals, losing almost 17 pounds, 4.5 inches and one dress size. And, of course, my relationship with the Lord has deepened!

What lies prevent you from moving toward the life that God wants for you? Are you ready to confront them? Here are a couple of lies that each of us needs to confront with the truth.

Confronting the Lies with Truth

Lie: *I am valued by how I look, what I wear and what I do.* We've heard this lie almost from the womb. The first time our mothers dressed us up in cute little outfits and we got praised; or when someone said, "Look at those cute little cheeks," we began to understand that our value was defined by the way others saw us. From those innocent, well-meaning comments to the outright attacks on our values by the media and our culture, we've been lied to our whole lives. Look good and people love you. Gain weight and be ignored.

Truth: *My value comes in knowing I am fully loved by God.* Allow these words to touch your heart and mind as you consider the truth of your worth: "How great is the love the Father has lavished on us, that we should be called children of God! And that is what we are!" (1 John 3:1).

As someone who has said yes to Jesus Christ as your ultimate guide and shepherd, you are no longer defined by what the world says, thinks or believes about you. You are a child of God! God literally lavishes you with love. He covers you with love. God does not see your body or your house or your car; He sees you and He says, "I love you!" In fact, God loves you so much that He was willing to give everything so that you could be with Him. You didn't have to do a thing.

Where did we get this idea that the more we weigh, the less valuable we are to God? Our culture has many negative preconceived notions about overweight people. Others judge us, and we judge ourselves. I have seen it over and over.

On the first night of a First Place 4 Health class when we all weigh in, I can see fear on the faces of those who come in the door. Some have not weighed themselves in years and have no idea how out of control their weight is. Others weigh themselves every day and know to the ounce how much they weigh. In either case, like my niece Abby, we allow the scale to define us and have power over us. We let the things in life—what happen to us, how we look, the kind of car we drive, the kind of job we have, and so on—determine our value. One of the many things that sets First Place 4 Health apart from other weight-loss programs is that it tells the truth. As I continue to study God's Word, I have come to understand that it is my relationship with God, not what I weigh, that defines who I am. I have had to have my mind totally changed and transformed by God's Word.

It's time for you to confront the lies and begin each day by saying, "I am a child of God and I am loved. God determines my worth, not the scale or even my own view of myself."

Lie: It is too hard for me to commit to anything: I am too busy and I don't have time. Too often we see our past failures and say, "I just can't commit." We believe the lie that "busy" means "purpose," when sometimes "busy" just means "busy." I heard a pastor once say that busy is just another way the devil keeps us from pursuing God's best. Busy may be defined as an acronym: Being Under Satan's Yoke. God has given us all the time we need to live a full life, if we simply reject the lie of the one who wants to destroy our wellbeing.

Truth: *When we commit our plans to God, He is more than able to work with us to see them through.* I love this passage from Psalm 3: "Commit your way to the LORD, trust in him and he will do this" (v. 5).

When we place our lives in God's hands and follow His plan, we are more than able to do what we need to do to experience a full life. As we commit time in the morning to prayer and a study of God's Word, God literally expands our days.

You will find time to do things that you never thought you had time to do! One of the hardest things I had to do when I began to follow God's plan for me was to wake up early for prayer and Bible study. I like sleep. No, let me rephrase that: I love sleep. With four kids, sleep was an elusive gift. I found that God gave me an even greater gift—time. When I gave my time to God, God gave that time right back to me! I was able to accomplish even more and felt more refreshed when I started my days in prayer and God's Word. Once I was in God's Word and feeling refreshed, I approached exercise with a whole new attitude. My heart was ready to receive the full life that God had for me. The scale lost its power, because I spent more time looking at God than at numbers. The same can happen for you!

Lie: I am not good at making wise decisions. The longer we are overweight, the more we believe this lie. The more diets we try and fail, the more we believe this lie. With every disapproving look from a parent, spouse or co-worker, we believe this lie. Every time we look in a mirror, we believe this lie. Having made unwise choices or decisions in the past does not determine what you can do today. With God's help, you can become one of the wisest people in the world!

Truth: *Our wisdom comes from God, and He's waiting for us to follow Him.* Solomon lived a long life and made many wise and foolish decisions. God gave him everything, but his desire for women took priority—at one point he had 700 wives and 300 concubines! Talk about an unwise decision! Like you, in his heart he wanted to follow God, but his desires pulled him away.

Solomon learned a simple truth: Wisdom comes in following God's plans, not your own. At one point in his life, Solomon wrote: "Trust in the LORD with all of your heart and lean not on your own understanding; in all your ways acknowledge him, and he will make your paths straight" (Prov. 3:5-6).

Because of his mistakes, Solomon learned that following God gave him the wisdom he needed to go down the right path. You do not have to be wise: God's wisdom can be yours. Your past mistakes will become God's building blocks. As you become healthier, you will bring glory to God. Join me in choosing to believe the wonderful truth that God will help us make wise decisions.

Lie: *I can't understand God.* So many people come to First Place 4 Health without having spent much time in prayer and Scripture. When I talk about knowing God and understanding His view, many new members quickly get discouraged because the few times they looked at the Bible, they got confused. They tried to read it once but they gave up, saying, "I can't understand God." Much like the high school student who believes that he or she will never understand algebra, we often give up too soon.

Truth: *With the help of the Holy Spirit and the Bible, I can better understand God.* Just like that high school student who could not understand algebra, you need help. I've got great news for you: God has already sent the greatest tutor in the universe—the Holy Spirit. Knowing that we would need help to understand God, Jesus said that after He left, God would send a Counselor to help us understand God's work (see John 14:16). The Greek word Jesus used to describe the Holy Spirit is *paraclete,* which literally means "one who is called to come alongside." In other words, God has promised to come alongside you to help you know and understand Him. You are not alone.

In addition to the Holy Spirit, we've also been given God's own words in the Bible. "All Scripture is God-breathed and is useful for teaching, rebuking, correcting and training in righteousness, so that the man of God may be thoroughly equipped for every good work" (2 Tim. 3:16-17). God has given us a manual to help us understand Him!

Whenever I hear the lie about not being able to understand God, I hold on to these powerful words from 1 Corinthians: "For who has known the mind of the Lord that he may instruct him? But we have the mind of Christ" (1 Cor. 2:16). We can literally have the mind of Christ!

When we start learning the truth, believing the truth and living in the truth, change will come. God wants us to believe Him. He can change any and every part of us: body, mind, emotions and spirit. What God really wants is for us to join Him in the transformation process—to participate and do our part! A great beginning place for us is to *stop believing the lies*!

Where the Lies Come From

In addition to knowing how to confront the lies with truth, it's helpful to know where the lies come from. Knowing the source of the lies not only removes their power but also increases our ability to do battle. Where do these lies come from? Three places: ourselves, the enemy of our souls, and the world.

Lies We Tell

First and foremost, we lie to ourselves. I once saw a Reebok store sign that read, "There is an athlete in all of us," and I believe it.

But most of us believe that there is no hope we can exercise, let alone become an athlete. Over the years, I have heard every imaginable excuse for not exercising. Here are just a few that I have heard. I promise that every one is genuine (I could not make this stuff up!):

- It's too hot.
- It's too cold.
- I'm too tired.
- I'm too busy.
- I feel faint when I walk.
- My throat hurts.
- My knee hurts.
- My feet hurt.
- I have to do laundry.
- My dog is sick.
- My husband is sick.
- I'm too old.
- I'm too stressed.
- I don't have any shoes.
- I don't have any money.
- I don't like people watching me.
- No one will go with me.
- I have to cook supper for my husband.
- I need to get my nails done.
- I have papers to grade.
- I have to clean my house.
- I don't want to build up my legs.
- My fat wiggles when I run.
- It shoots my morning.
- It shoots my evening.
- I'll miss *CSI*.
- I need to work.
- I have homework.
- I have my grandchildren.
- Exercise doesn't work for me; it runs in my family.

- It's so boring.
- I don't like sweating.
- I get nauseated.
- I can't get up.
- It ruins my hair.
- My thyroid won't let me.
- My trainer hates me.

I believe that if you really want to do something, you will find the motivation to do it. You need to stop lying to yourself. It is not too cold, it is not too hot, and your trainer does not hate you. Stop lying to yourself and at least be honest. You do not want to exercise. I am not going to try to convince you that if you start exercising, you will learn to love it. That is not necessarily true for everyone. I can say that if you are consistent with your commitment you will start experiencing the benefits and you will at least be able to tolerate your exercise routine.

There are other lies we tell ourselves as well, such as the lie that if we do more, God will love us more. This was a lie with which I had to contend in my own life.

I do not consider myself a runner. My definition of a runner is someone who can run a mile in 8 minutes or less, not 15 minutes. I am a slow jogger—a *slogger*, to be exact. Several years ago, I decided to run a marathon. I had been jogging about 20 miles a week and thought I was up to the challenge. I shared with a group of my close friends (boasting in the form of a prayer request) that one of my goals was to run a marathon. They were all so excited and extremely supportive, encouraging me to go for it and assuring me that I could do it. Some of those who had actually completed a marathon themselves said it would be the "ultimate spiritual experience." I was pumped! These people were going to be so proud of me!

I trained everywhere I could as much as I could, even while on vacation in North Carolina. I was running through beautiful mountains one afternoon and I found myself praying, "Lord, I can just feel You giving me strength. I am going to do this! It's going to be so great! You are going to be so proud of me!"

I did indeed feel His Spirit. It was one of those times when He comes in His gentle way and invades your mind, leaving you with no doubt it's a thought from Him.

He clearly said to me, "Yes, Vicki, this is a wonderful thing. And I will have something to tell you when you cross that finish line. In fact, it is so profound that I am going to tell you right now." I stopped in my tracks. I stopped running and just waited to absorb this message from the Lord.

He said, "I am going to tell you when you cross that finish line that *I won't love you anymore than I do right now.*" Wow, once again I had been sucked into believing the lie that if I did more and tried harder, God would love me more. I thought that if I ran a marathon, He would love me more! When will I ever learn to recognize the lies that come from within? The truth is that the God of the universe loves me just as I am right now. It is the *truth.*

It's not about what you can do or what you feel like you have to keep trying to do; it's about what God can do and what He has already done for you. He loves you just as you are today and will never love you more than He does today. Accept it and believe it.

Lies Satan Tells

The enemy of your soul, Satan, will also lie to you. One of Satan's biggest lies is that you cannot change. You will fail. Whatever you do will make no difference. Satan wants to rob you of the joy of success. He wants to rob you of the life that God has planned for you. If he can keep you on the couch, he will keep you in the pit. Satan will use whatever He can to draw you away from God. From the very beginning, the devil has been trying to pull us away from God's best for our lives.

I recently talked with a lady who truly believes that she cannot exercise. She called about the classes I teach, saying that she was just curious. She shared with me that she has never been successful at any kind of exercise. I invited her to just try one of my classes and then give me her honest opinion. She had a great time! Part of her success was the fellowship she experienced by walking into a faith-based exercise class. They do exist!

Lies the World Tells

Finally, the world and all of its so-called common sense lies to us. The world says that we will never be able to reach our goals and there is nothing wrong with taking it easy. Common sense says that a woman in her fifties cannot teach a boot camp twice a week and that a grandmother is supposed to be "fluffy." What I know to be the truth is that my God is not a common God. On the contrary, He takes common ordinary people and does uncommon things with them. About three years ago, I started developing a boot-camp program for Body and Soul Fitness, and I have been teaching those classes ever since. We serve an uncommon God.

What You Need to Do

Are there lies that you have believed that need to be replaced with God's truth? Ask God to give you His truth as a replacement for every lie you have believed. And begin to learn to confront the sources of these lies. As you start believing and living out the truth, change will come. I want you to look forward to what God is going to do. I expect Him to be faithful, and He has never let me down. God won't let you down either.

A New Way of Thinking

I became a Christian at the age of 18. While I had some positive influences in my life before that, my first 18 years were not filled with God's voice but with other voices that influenced my entire view of the world. As a result, as a new Christian I had a lot of negative thinking to overcome. I had been exposed to a lot of criticism growing up, all of which impacted the way I saw the world and viewed myself.

One of the tapes that has played over and over in my memory is a recording of my mom telling me, "If you eat that, you're going to get fat," and "Don't wear that shirt—it makes you look bigger." The first thing my mom ever noticed about someone was the way he or she looked. As a result of hearing criticism of myself and others for most of my life, I had come to believe that the outside of a person was what counted. As you can imagine, I did not have a perfect body growing up, and I always felt ashamed of the way I looked. I paid constant attention to my weight and appearance and felt I had to strive for perfection. Even after I became a Christian, these ideas occasionally still rose to the surface.

In addition to the criticism that I grew up hearing and believing, I incorporated some bad theology in my life. Sometimes churches teach wrong ideas, and sometimes we just pick them up on our own. But one way or the other, I had become a young adult who spent years striving to please God by being perfect. I just knew that God would only be pleased with me if I had perfect attendance at church, went on every youth trip and memorized all my Bible verses.

Satan would use those thoughts and the memories of things I had done in my past to remind me that I was not worthy to be leading, teaching or doing much at all for the Lord. Then one day I realized that I had to do something drastic about my thoughts. When lies become deeply rooted in our pattern of thinking, we need to dig deep to pull out the roots, because our minds—how we think—are central to the way we view ourselves and our behaviors.

God wants to transform a depraved mind (and, sadly, all of us have depraved minds due to sin) into one that is controlled by the Holy Spirit. This condition of the mind is what Paul referred to in Romans 8:6, where he states, "The mind of sinful man is death, but the mind controlled by the Spirit is life and peace." We have a choice in the way we behave, because we have a choice in the way we think. If the Spirit is influencing our thinking, our behavior will change!

Like a Tree Planted by a River

I began to change my thinking with Scripture. I started reading God's Word, meditating on it and memorizing it. Slowly, God began to replace my negative thinking with His words. A transformation began in my life as God's words confronted the lies that had become such a deeply rooted part of me. You see, God is in the business of mind control. When we allow God's words to have priority in our lives, we develop the ability to control our thinking and take every thought captive: "We take captive every thought to make it obedient to Christ" (1 Cor. 10:5). God's Word has the power to replace negative thinking with the truth.

I remember so clearly when this renewing process actually began to take effect. I was teaching Sunday School and talking about God's love when suddenly a memory of something I had done years ago came flooding back. Satan was there, pointing his bony accusing finger at me. The funny thing was that the images were no longer in living color. They had actually faded to black and white and were barely visible. He no longer had power over me. God's truth had transformed my mind! God's spirit now had control over my thoughts! I almost laughed out loud!

Psalm 1 begins:

Blessed is the man who does not walk in the counsel of the wicked or stand in the way of sinners or sit in the seat of mockers. But his delight is in the law of the LORD, and on his law he meditates day and night (vv. 1-2).

You will be blessed, or find happiness, when you choose to allow God's words to take the place of all the negative voices from your past that are trying to keep you down. In fact, you will be "like a tree planted by streams of water, which yields its fruit in season and whose leaf does not wither. Whatever [you do] prospers" (Ps. 1:3). When we allow God's words to take hold, we'll begin to see positive results! Because I planted myself deep in God's words, His water gave me a new outlook on myself and on God's ability to work through me.

Do you want to begin the process of changing your mind? Begin each day with Scripture. Each day I read one chapter from the Old Testament and then a chapter from the New Testament. If reading two chapters a day seems like a lot right now, read one chapter. If that feels like a lot, begin with a verse or two.

As you become more familiar with God's Word, you will want to start memorizing verses from it. You may even want to start with Psalm 1 and memorize that amazing promise. At the end of this book, I've included an appendix of some Scripture verses to memorize and have ready for times when Satan tries to lead you astray. Whatever you do, begin today and enjoy the fruits of a changed mind.

A Warning

By itself, knowing or reading God's Word does not guarantee success. You also need to put it into action and walk by the faith that is growing in you. Listen to this powerful story:

At the village church in Kalonovka, Russia, attendance at Sunday school picked up after the priest started handing out candy to the peasant children. One of the most faithful was a pug-nosed, pugnacious lad who recited his Scriptures with proper piety, pocketed his reward, and then fled into the fields to eat it.

The priest took a liking to the boy, persuading him to attend church school. This was preferable to doing household chores from which his devout parents excused him. By offering other inducements, the priest managed to teach the boy the four Gospels. In fact, the boy won a special prize for learning all four by heart and reciting them nonstop in church. Now, 60 years later, he still likes to recite Scriptures, but in a context that would horrify the old priest. For the prize pupil, who memorized so much of the Bible, is Nikita Khrushchev, the former Communist czar.

As this anecdote illustrates, the "why" behind memorization is as important as the "what." The same Nikita Khrushchev who nimbly mouthed God's Word as a child, later declared God to be nonexistent—because his cosmonauts had not seen Him. Khrushchev memorized the Scriptures for the candy, the rewards and the bribes, rather than for the meaning it had for his life.[1]

We do not simply need to know God's Word—we need to apply it to our lives and allow it to change our hearts and our behaviors. I realized early on that if I continued to sin, I would provide Satan with more ways to accuse me. Now I try to be quick to obey and quick to confess when I realize I have sinned against God. I do not let sin take root in my mind. This transformed thinking has had a direct impact on my values and behavior.

The same thing can be true in regard to our thoughts about being a fit and healthy person. So many of us need to change our minds about what it really means to be a fit and healthy person. If we can replace old, misleading thinking with new, accurate thinking, our actions will follow suit and our behaviors will change. Failure will no longer be a warm and familiar friend.

Our behaviors will take on a new consistency, and we will start to experience success. This process takes time and will not happen overnight. But the most important part of the process is for you to actually start.

A Paradigm Shift

A paradigm shift is a radical change in our understanding of the world. Paradigm shifts happen in all areas of our lives. One might say that to become a Christian, you undergo the ultimate paradigm shift. All things become new. Paul said it this way: "If anyone is in Christ, he is a new creation; the old has gone, the new has come!" (2 Cor. 5:17). In other words, God changes the way we understand and view the world. He is ever working in our minds and hearts to transform our thinking by the power of His Word and the influence of His Holy Spirit.

Over the past 10 years, a paradigm shift has been happening in the wellness industry. A new generation of researchers, physicians and health-promotion specialists are working diligently to change our views of health, exercise and weight. This new paradigm debunks some of the old ways of thinking and gives us a new way to view the world and ourselves. God is all about change, so let's see where we need to change our minds about several long-held ways of thinking about wellness.

Wrong Thinking: *Thin Means Healthy*

At the very base of this new wellness paradigm is a change in one of the assumptions that we have held for many years. For most of the twentieth century, people have believed that being thin ensures both good health and happiness. "You can't be too thin," an expression we have heard for years, implies that the thinner you are, the more valuable and superior you are—a supposition that simply is not true. Physiologically it may not be true either. There are many people who are very thin, but have extremely poor eating habits, which in turn cause high cholesterol and other problems and deficiencies.

Wrong Thinking: *Overweight People Lack Willpower*

Society in general assumes that people who are not thin lack will-power and either eat too much or are too lazy to exercise. The assumed solution to being overweight, then, is to simply eat less and exercise more. We wish it were that simple! We know that simply dieting alone rarely works, because this leads to the yo-yo effect: We lose the weight while on the diet and regain it as soon as we return to our old patterns. Physicians and weight researchers also recognize there are genetic factors and physiological mechanisms that play a part in determining body shape and size—and a person's ability to shed extra pounds.

Right Thinking: *Wellness Is Not Just About Weight*

We need to have our minds transformed to a new way of thinking and get rid of the old faulty assumptions. The old way of thinking says that it's all about size, but really it's all about health.

A much better approach to being healthy would be to focus on things other than weight loss: healthy eating, regular exercise, positive self-esteem and, perhaps most importantly, an understanding of who you are in Christ, which will have a huge impact on self-acceptance. Being healthy has less to do with a number on a scale than the ability to balance and embrace all aspects of one's life: the emotional, mental and spiritual, as well as the physical.

You'll have your own paradigm shift toward your wellness goals as you identify old patterns of thought that are destructive and replace them with new thoughts that will propel you toward your goals.

Out with the Old Thinking, in with the New

I love the way Paul encouraged the congregation in Philippi to replace their old ways of thinking with God's perspective on what's good in the world. In Philippians 4:8, he says, "Brothers, whatever is true, whatever is noble, whatever is right, whatever is pure, whatever is lovely, whatever is admirable—if anything is excellent or praiseworthy—think about such things." He challenges the believers to see and think differently. Every Christian needs to embrace God's perspective on the world. Let's look at some old ways of thinking about body image, exercise, health and eating, and replace those old views with new ways to look at our lives.

Old thinking: *Exercise is a form of punishment for having an imperfect body.* Is this what you believe about exercise? So often people approach their workout sessions with fear and dread, because they know just how tired they'll be in the middle of them. Some people even exercise to punish themselves for overeating. I actually had one lady say to me as she came into class, "Work me hard today—I have been bad." "No pain, no gain" has become a proverb for the health industry. But when our thinking begins with shame or includes the word "pain," it's no wonder that most of us don't want to get out of bed to exercise!

New thinking: *I can be thankful for the opportunity to exercise.* What would happen if we began by thinking about the gain and the privilege of exercise? This has been a huge change for me. Below, I've listed five reasons that I am thankful for exercise. You might want to use some of these to help change your own way of thinking:

- *Thanksgiving #1: It's made my heart strong.* At the age of 56, my father suffered his first heart attack. That age is only five years away for me, but according to my doctor and my most recent medical exam, I have "practically wiped out my chances" of coronary heart disease because of my active lifestyle! Even a small amount of exercise is better than none, and more is better than less.

- *Thanksgiving #2: It's helped me stand up straight!* Being a small-boned person, I am at a higher risk than most people of developing osteoporosis as I age. Exercise, together with a healthy calcium (with vitamin D) intake, builds strong bones. I stand taller and feel better about myself, and I give thanks!

• *Thanksgiving #3: It's kept me from losing my mind!* For years I exercised for vanity, but now I exercise for sanity! Exercise is God's natural antidepressant for the body. There have been many times in my life that I have been burdened with problems and the cares of this world and have headed out the door to get outside, enjoy the fresh air and sunshine, and have been able to come home with a much better outlook on whatever problems are plaguing me. Exercise gives my mind a whole new perspective on my day.

• *Thanksgiving #4: It's helped me have four healthy pregnancies.* Although exercise might be risky for some pregnant women, the benefits of exercising during pregnancy generally far outweigh the risks. During all four of my pregnancies, I was able to exercise almost up to the last trimester. During my last pregnancy, I walked the same route every morning with two of my dear friends, making friends along the way, including a sweet elderly gentleman. One morning he just couldn't resist saying, "You girls are sure working hard. And it seems to be working for two of you, but that one in the middle just keeps getting bigger and bigger!"

• *Thanksgiving #5: It's given me fitness friends!* Over the years, exercise has introduced me to some of the most outstanding athletes in the world! I have made friends all over the country, because of the opportunities I've had to speak about exercise. I have walking buddies in Ohio; kayaking friends in Mississippi; running buddies in Texas; aerobic friends in Nairobi, Kenya; dancing friends in DC; and weight-lifting friends at Cathedral of Praise!

Exercise has truly enriched my life in more ways than one! I am thankful everyday that I *get* to exercise, not that I *have* to!

When you exercise regularly, you will feel better. It's a fact. When you take the time to walk, run, lift, push and pull, your body will thank you for it. You'll have more energy and better health for a lifetime. Focus on that fact. When the alarm goes off in the morning, your first thought about exercise should be, *I'm going to feel so good after I exercise!*

Old thinking: I am sad, so what can I eat? In chapter 8, we'll talk more about our relationship with food, but for now let me say this: *Food is not your counselor.* God provided food to bring us comfort through nourishment, so in a sense every type of food is comfort food, but food is not the ultimate comforter. Food cannot provide us with help or love or support or assistance. Food cannot solve our problems or walk with us through them. Food might be able to numb us temporarily, but the pain or sadness will inevitably return.

New thinking: I am sad, so who can I call? God's greatest gifts are people who love and support you, and prayer. Whether or not the person you call is on the same road to wellness as you, you will find that calling a friend, pastor or family member will do more to bless you in your sadness than a pint of ice cream. Prayer and crying out to God can also be a wonderful response to sadness. Sometimes I have to sing to God at the top of my lungs to get me out of the pit and my feet back on solid ground.

Old thinking: I am bored, so what can I eat? Let's be honest: We've all eaten out of boredom. We feel as if not much is happening in our lives, so we decide to do something—anything—and we head for the bag of chips or the box of cookies. Or if we don't want to start a project or get to work, we delay being productive by convincing ourselves that we are hungry. One of the worst things about eating while feeling bored is that we are likely to consume many more calories than we really need. A great example is the new fourth meal. This is a meal that is being marketed as the meal you eat round 10 o'clock at night (because we are open 24 hours!), when you are still up and have nothing else to do.

New thinking: I am bored, so what can I do? Choose to do something productive—even something small. Choose a project that you wish you had time for, and every time you are tempted to eat when you're not hungry, work on the project for 10 or 15 minutes. You'll experience two wonderful benefits: (1) You'll be keeping the weight off, and (2) you'll enjoy the results of your labor. Jesus said it so well: "If anyone would come after me, he must deny himself and *take up his cross daily* and follow me" (Luke 9:23, emphasis added). That second step, "take up his cross," indicates finding a redemptive ministry and doing it. One of my redemptive ministries is teaching: I teach Bible study and fitness classes. When I am bored, God's spirit brings me back to my redemptive ministries, and there is always something I can do to prepare for the next class.

Old thinking: *I should focus on what I can't have.* One of Satan's oldest tricks is to get us to focus on what we can't have. Way back in the Garden, he pointed out what Adam and Eve couldn't eat. If we do the same thing, we'll always feel left out and discouraged, and we'll pay the price of a lifetime of ill health.

New thinking: *I should focus on the abundance of good food choices that I have.* God's abundance is extraordinary, and the choices we're given are almost limitless, so why complain about not being able to eat a particular food? Imagine the endless combinations of food available at a farmer's market or in the produce section of your local grocery store! Our Father in heaven knows what we need, and He's made an endless variety of food just for us. We live in the most affluent country in the world and have almost everything we need for delicious healthy meals right at our fingertips. And the Internet has tons of websites with great recipes and meal-planning suggestions.

Out with the Old Behaviors, in with the New

As these new and healthy patterns of thinking take root in our minds, our behaviors start to change. We *do* have a choice about how we think and live. And this transforming of our minds with new thinking is about more than just positive thinking. God's Word says that He will move us beyond just the positive (see Phil. 4:13)!

Although the Bible provides a way to transform our way of thinking, some effort on our part *is* required. In Ephesians 3:20, Paul states, "Now to him who is able to do immeasurably more than all we ask or imagine, according to his power that is at work within us, to him be glory."

So many people approach weight loss backwards. They begin with behavior: They make their bodies participate in exercises that they really don't want to do. They make their bodies go on a diet and deny themselves foods that are nutritious if eaten in proper portions. Then they hope they will think about themselves differently and eventually have a new mindset. The approach is as follows:

change behavior = hopeful thinking = new mindset

Let me tell you right now that this approach will not work. How many people have you known who have decided to get fit and then went on a diet, exercised like crazy, lost weight and then gained it all back? We see this going on all around us. The problem is that there was only a temporary change in behavior and not a permanent change in thinking.

God's paradigm is just the opposite. We first change our mindset, allowing God to have first place in our lives. God takes our thoughts and attitudes and begins to shape them into His image, helping us change our thinking. We replace the old ways of thinking with new, healthier ways of thinking. Only then do we begin to change our behaviors into ones that we can walk in for a lifetime.

A new mind *equals* a new way of thinking, which *equals* new behavior:

new mindset = new thinking = changed behaviors

Your new ways of behaving will stay with you because they do not have to battle an old mindset. You'll have a new paradigm to health and wellness! Let me give you a few examples of a new mindset that led to new thinking, which in turn led to changed behaviors in my own life.

Old behavior: *Speed eating.* Eating quickly reminds me of lunchtime during school. You only have 15 minutes to wolf your lunch down and get to your locker. The truth is that this is rarely the situation any of us find ourselves in.

New behavior: *Eating slowly.* Someone once said, "Why eat when you can dine?" Eating too fast undermines healthy digestion and encourages overeating. When we eat our meals too quickly, we don't give our bodies time to send and receive the signals that we have had enough. When we hurry our eating, we also tend to miss the sensory aspects of food: the smell of it, the way the food looks, even the taste of what we're eating. Paying attention to our food always helps us avoid mindless eating. We all have experienced that shocking moment when we've looked down at an empty potato chip bag and said to ourselves, *Who ate that?*

Old behavior: *Overfeeding my body.* The average American overfeeds his or her body by approximately 30 percent! We consume more than we actually need for a plethora of reasons. In a recent study done by a major university, 100 college students were told to go through a cafeteria line, choosing anything they wanted. After sitting down at the table, they were to remove one third of each item chosen and consume the rest. They all lost weight!

New behavior: *Accepting less as more.* According to Lisa Young, author of *The Portion Teller: Smartsize Your Way to Permanent Weight Loss,* neither carbs nor fats are to blame for America's obesity problem. It's the volume.[2] "Super Size My Thighs" should be the slogan of some restaurant chains! I remember watching a Food Network show with an American chef competing against a Japanese chef to produce the most savory meal. Both chefs came up with equally beautiful meals, and the American chef pointed out the similarities in the quality of both meals. The Japanese chef, however, pointed out one glaring difference between the two: The American meal was large enough to feed an entire Japanese family.

As you consider what new behavior and thinking you want to add to your life, read Sarah's story. As she spent time with her heavenly Dad, He slowly began to change her thinking and motivate her behavior:

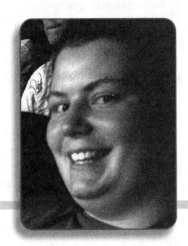 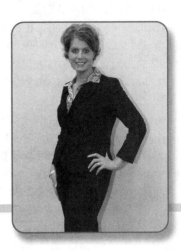

SARAH MIELKE

It was supposed to be hereditary. I would struggle with weight my whole life. I was "big boned" and would have to be content with having a pretty face. I had surrendered to that fact, until I decided to give God first place in every area of my life: mental, spiritual, emotional and physical.

Although I'd grown up in a Baptist preacher's home and at a very young age had trusted the Lord for salvation, I just couldn't seem to control my eating. Even as a type-A control freak, I couldn't get a hold of the only thing that I could truly control—myself.

My health became a concern to my family. I couldn't fit into clothes at the department store, and my grandmother offered me $500 to lose 20 pounds (which my parents agreed to match!). Toward the end of my high school years, I was only able to shop in plus-size stores. But it was hereditary. I was big boned. And I had a pretty face.

Vocationally, I had decided to follow in my parents' path. I wanted to serve in full-time ministry in a local church, and I went to a private Baptist college for my undergraduate work. I wanted to tell others about my relationship with God and how He could change their lives. But would they listen to me when it was so obvious that I was not disciplined? How could I convince them to let God change their lives if I didn't let Him change mine? According to the health professionals, I was considered extremely morbidly obese.

I began to understand that I was designed as a unique person by the Creator, and He had a wonderful plan for my life. Although this was something I had known for years, I finally began to embrace the concept. My dad and I began to have conversations about my life and my weight. He was not condescending nor did he plead with me to change; he just explained that I was a four-sided person and that God wanted to work in my mental, emotional and physical life, not just the spiritual.

When I discovered the First Place 4 Health program, it was exactly what I needed. Not a diet plan, First Place 4 Health wasn't only about the weight. Different from other weight-loss and fitness programs, we use a Live It Tracker to record what we eat and our fitness activity. The title of our tracker embraces the notion that we can have new *life* in Christ. See how that thinking is different from a "*die*-it"?

I wrote down everything I ate, renewed my commitment to daily Bible reading and began to exercise every day. Setting small goals, I began to achieve them. Looking at each decision through the lens of obedience, I worked toward bringing God glory, and the weight began to fall off.

The First Place 4 Health program elements have been crucial in my weight loss, my relationship with the Lord and others, and my learning how to walk daily with God. It's all about balance and honoring the Lord with my heart, soul, mind and strength. Each day, each moment, I have the opportunity to experience victory and joy!

Does it sound like First Place 4 Health is a lot to do? I'm also managing the daily organization of my home, working full-time and writing the dissertation for my doctorate. If *I* have time, so do *you*.

I lost most of the weight in two years, and I have kept it off for over five years. I've also completed four half-marathons.

Unlike other programs, the First Place 4 Health program is not a quick fix. It's not a program to go on until you lose weight and then go off of once you've achieved a magical number on a scale. This is a lifestyle of health and a faith journey. It's a new way of life that I will continue, because I will always need the balance in my life, regardless of what number appears on the scales.

Gone forever are 152 pounds! Looks like someone owes me $1,000! *Soli Deo gloria!*

Old behavior: *Needing to eat something sweet.* One of my favorite indulgences is chocolate. A small amount of chocolate can be good for you, particularly dark chocolate, which is full of antioxidants. My problem is that I want to eat the creamy milk chocolate found in a Snickers candy bar.

New behavior: *Cultivating the palate.* It's no surprise that we really love sweets. For many of us, dessert time was an important part of our day when we were growing up. One of my favorite sayings was "Save your fork—dessert is coming!" We seem to suffer from a sense of deprivation when we do not have sweets. But sugary foods can overwhelm our taste buds and dull our senses. One of the simplest changes I made to my behavior in this regard was to substitute an individually wrapped sweet prune for the candy bar. The prune satisfies my craving for something sweet and is also a fiber-rich healthy snack. The point is that a healthy food plan can still be full of wonderful treats. Redefine dessert, and you will be amazed at how naturally sweet fruits are.

When we allow our thinking to be transformed by the Holy Spirit and God's Word, our behaviors *can* be changed. It will be hard work, but God promises to help you with the process. Wellness *will* happen, "for God is working in you, giving you the desire and the power to do what pleases him" (Phil. 2:13, *NLT*).

You can resist, you can run, but God has set a goal for you: to be transformed into the image of His Son—and He is not giving up on you.

4

Obstacles and Ways to Overcome Them

When my children were young and January 1 came around, one of them always asked me, "Mom, are you going to make any New Year's revolutions?" Maybe "revolution" is actually a better word than "resolution." Whether you are choosing to make a revolution or a resolution, both words are indicative of change.

In 1968, there was a song by the Beatles called "Revolution" that a few of you may remember. It was on the B-side of a very popular single called "Hey Jude." (A long, long time ago, music was released on these little round disks called records.) John Lennon wrote it while in India at a transcendental meditation camp with the Maharishi, and it begins with the words:

You say you want a revolution.
Well, you know,
We all want to change the world.

What you may have discovered along with the Beatles is that we have very limited power on our own to change anything—ourselves or the world.

Have you ever had this experience? On January 1, you pull out your new exercise clothes (you picked them up while in the stores, exchanging your Christmas gifts) and maybe even break open a new exercise DVD by the latest Hollywood weight-loss guru. Excited to use your new gym membership, you wake up at 6 AM on January 2 so you can be there when the doors open. You proudly eat half a banana and a bowl of yogurt, feeling confident and inspired to jump-start your newly formed "eating less and moving more" action plan.

The first week you do pretty well, and you are amazed at how good you feel. *I should have been doing this my whole life,* you proudly think to yourself. At the beginning of the second week, you begin to feel a little bit of pain, because you've pushed it too hard the first week, and running on the treadmill (which was so exciting the first five days) has become a little boring. By the middle of the second week, you find that it's getting harder to get up to exercise in the morning, because you've got a little too much to do.

By day 14, you step on the scale and realize that while you lost two or three pounds the first week, you've now actually gained back a pound. Feeling discouraged and deflated, you take the next two days off. By day three of the third week, you wonder why you even started.

If this sounds familiar, you are not alone.

Do you realize that by January 17, most people have given up on their New Year's resolutions to get healthy? That date has practically become recognized as an official holiday. Amazing! Are we really that pitiful? Eight out of 10 people will give up their resolve from the New Year within the first three weeks. Most of us just don't have it in us to push through the obstacles that come our way.

However, you can break the pattern. With the new way of thinking that is taking place in you right now, there is hope that you will no longer be the average person who quits his or her wellness endeavors after just a few weeks but will be well above average! You know the truth, and the truth is that you can do all things through Christ who gives you strength (see Phil. 4:13)!

Jesus is the secret to sticking with your wellness plan, so let's look at the four obstacles to exercise most people run into and deal with them right now.

Obstacle #1: Time Constraints

We are a busy and exhausted people. As a full-time pastor's wife, mother of four, writer and speaker, I've had my share of extremely demanding days. But I learned early on that if I were not intentional, my days would be consumed with activity that seemed urgent in the moment but had no long-lasting benefit to my life or the lives of those I loved.

Whenever I'm tempted to feel like a victim to the demands on my time, I remember the life of Jesus. If anyone was busy, it was Jesus. The more popular He became, the more things He had to do. In fact, one day as He was getting off a boat after crossing the Sea of Galilee, a huge crowd swarmed Him with their needs and concerns. One man's needs trumped them all, however. Jairus, a ruler in the synagogue, got Jesus' attention because his daughter was dying. Jesus' heart was moved by this father, who pleaded desperately at His feet.

As Jesus made His way through the crowd, everyone wanted a piece of Him, almost literally. The crowds were grabbing Him, begging Him, asking Him to pay attention to them. (Every mom who stays at home with small children knows this feeling!) Jesus didn't flinch, though, because He knew His mission at that moment: to save Jairus's daughter. He didn't flinch, until a woman who had been bleeding for 12 years touched His robe. Suddenly, everything stopped. Jesus wanted to discover who had touched Him, so that He could encourage the woman who was healed. I find this amazing. Jairus pleaded with Jesus to hurry, the crowds begged Him for attention, and yet Jesus controlled the situation and looked for the woman. Finding her, He blessed her, and only then did He move on.

How was Jesus able to do that? Instead of being a victim to time, Jesus knew that God had everything under control, so He was free to pursue God's best. Events were not given the power to control Him, because He knew that God had control of the events.

The truth is that we control our time—we choose how to spend the time God gives us. Time is only a series of events, and when we control the events, we can control our time. Time is one of our most valuable commodities. Becoming healthy will definitely cost us something, and aside from costing us money and energy, it will cost us some of our time. But what we spend will be well worth the investment.

When Jesus stopped to heal the woman, it also cost something: Jairus's daughter died. But God had a larger plan—the girl would be raised from the dead! What Jesus lost at the beginning, He gained at the end.

The same holds true for you. As you seek to honor God in caring for your body and pursuing His best, you'll find that He will abundantly provide the time, money and energy you need to reach your goals. We worship an amazing God who is more than able to supply our needs as we place Him first in our lives.

One way to begin to control your time and set priorities for a better way to live is to take it one step at a time, literally. What defeats a lot of us from the beginning is the thinking that getting fit will cost us at least an hour each day to work out. We imagine that exercising is something huge and more time-consuming and complicated than it really is. We think that we have to spend energy convincing ourselves that we want and need to exercise and then we have to change clothes, find our gym shoes, drive to the gym, work out and then get back home.

Exercise simply does not have to be that complicated. What we fail to realize is that there are many ways to increase activity in our lives without programming it into an already jam-packed schedule. The simplest and least time-consuming way to increase your activity level is to increase your steps. You may not have time in your busy day to fit in an exercise class, but you can increase the number of steps you take as you go about your day-to-day activities. You'll experience tons of benefits by simply increasing the number of steps you take every day!

To do this, first determine your step baseline. Keep track of the number of steps you take in a typical day for three days, and then average the numbers to obtain your baseline. After doing this, use the following numbers to figure out your physical activity level (these numbers are for healthy adults):

- 5,000 steps a day may be used to indicate a sedentary lifestyle.
- 5,000-7,499 steps a day is typical of normal daily activity excluding sports and exercise and might be considered a low-active lifestyle.

- 7,500-9,999 steps a day likely includes some purposeful activities (and/or elevated occupational activity) and might be considered a somewhat active lifestyle.
- 10,000 steps a day indicates the point at which an individual could be classified as active.
- Individuals who take more that 12,500 steps a day are likely to be classified as highly active.[1]

In order to increase your activity level, gradually add 200 to 1,000 steps a day to your baseline, until you are walking 10,000 steps a day. Ten thousand steps are approximately five miles, so build up gradually. Finding one chunk of time to walk five miles a day would take at least an hour, but by increasing the number of steps you take little by little, you will not feel like you are giving up so much time.

How do you add steps? Here are a few simple ideas:

- Park your car in the parking spot that is the farthest from the door of whatever store you have to go into.
- Carry the laundry to the washer in two trips instead of piling it up and taking only one trip.
- Get up from your computer every half hour and walk around the room for a minute.
- Play music and dance around the kitchen while you put the clean dishes away.
- Gradually add a few minutes or a few blocks to any regular walking/jogging that you normally do.
- And of course, you can always take the dog out for a quick walk at lunchtime or when you first get home from work!

You will need to purchase a reliable pedometer. Pedometers are simple devices you can clip onto your clothes that count the number of steps you take. Tracking your steps by detecting body motion means that even small steps can help speed you toward your fitness goals. You may even discover that you'll get a little addicted to seeing just how many steps it takes to walk to the mailbox or down to the corner or to get into the car!

Pedometers are relatively inexpensive, but they may have more features than you actually need. So follow these simple guidelines:

- Choose a pedometer with a large display screen that is easy to read.
- Make sure the pedometer has a clip that stays snug against your body and won't slip or bounce off, and that it has a safety strap in case it does.
- Remember to wear your pedometer! Keep it in a prominent place, like on your shaving kit or make-up bag so that you will remember to put it on every morning.

In talking about the Christian life, Paul encouraged the church in Rome to "never be lacking in zeal, but keep your spiritual fervor, serving the Lord" (Rom. 12:11). I believe this applies to every aspect of our walk with Christ, including how we literally walk. As you become more zealous for God, allow God to literally increase your steps.

Walking 10,000 steps a day is a wonderful way to have an active lifestyle without having to program into your schedule a block of daily exercise time. Studies on benefits of 10,000 steps a day report the following:

- Increasing steps helps prevent heart disease in women. Heart disease is on the decline in men but increasing in women. Women are six times more likely to die from heart disease than breast cancer, and heart disease kills more women over 65 than any other disease.
- Pedometers encourage people to walk more. When you are watching your numbers each day, you make better choices about where you park your car or whether you take the stairs. The simple act of being aware will help you to become healthier quicker, even if you don't take 10,000 steps every day.[2]

- Middle-aged women who take at least 10,000 steps per day are much more likely to fall into the recommended ranges for measures of body composition such as total body weight and body fat percentage.[3] Inactive women who take fewer than 6,000 steps per day are more likely to be overweight or obese and have higher waist circumferences, a strong predictor of increased risk of cardiovascular disease.[4]

Speaking of time, ours will not go on forever. Let's be honest: Time in this life is a limited resource, and how we use it makes all the difference in our world. I love how the psalmist talks about the limits of our life in Psalm 90:10-12:

The length of our days is seventy years—or eighty, if we have strength; yet their span is but trouble and sorrow, for they quickly pass, and we fly away.... Teach us to number our days aright, that we may gain a heart of wisdom.

Although a genuine effort to increase our steps is a great way to increase the activity in our life and get over the obstacle of thinking that we don't have enough time, an even greater reason to deal with the issue of time is that some of us may be running out of it. We have the misguided belief that we have all the time in the world to get healthy, so we think we can afford to put fitness on our "tomorrow" list.

My mother was diagnosed with stage four lung cancer in the summer of 2009. She had been fairly active most of her life. She was a member of a mall-walker's club, she worked hard in her garden, and there were some days I could not keep up with her energy. She started slowing down little by little, and finally in the second year after my father's death, she gave up her healthy lifestyle. No longer meeting her friends at the mall for an early-morning walk, she also let the garden go and had someone else come by to do the necessary yard work.

By the time she was diagnosed with lung cancer, she had become very inactive. As we met with the doctor, I asked him what we could do to beat this cancer and if there was a cure. Unfortunately, neither chemotherapy nor radiation would have a positive effect on this kind of cancer. The only possible hope was the removal of the malignant lung, and even that had only a slim chance of success. My mom quickly told the doctor that she was willing to have the lung removed. He went on to tell her that not everyone is a candidate for this surgery. Brutal on the body, lung-removal surgery puts a huge strain on the heart. He asked, "Mrs. Hensley, can you walk a mile at a good strong pace?" She said she could not today, but she was willing to put in the time and effort to get her heart strong enough for the surgery. Sadly, he told us that it was too late for that. Her type of cancer would spread quickly in the next six months. My mom died less than a year later.

By contrast, consider what happened to Carole Lewis's mother, Francis Harper, who died when she was almost 90:

> It was the early 1990s and my mom had rented a beach house on Bolivar, just across the bay from Galveston Island. Our family had gathered to play for an entire week. On Saturday afternoon the guys were cooking on the grill and the women were sitting on the porch talking when my mom said that she wasn't feeling well. She went inside to lay down and kept feeling worse. I felt her forehead and it was really hot. The closest thing we had to a doctor was Johnny's brother, Mike (who is a dentist), so he came in to check on her and said he thought we needed to take her to the hospital.
>
> It seemed to take forever to get on the ferry and get to John Sealy Hospital in Galveston. Once we got there, Mom sat in a wheelchair all night, waiting for a room in the emergency department. By the time they checked her over, she was running a high fever and was deathly sick.
>
> After being admitted to a room, she was diagnosed with streptococcal septicemia. We were grateful to be at John Sealy, a teaching hospital, because my mom got wonderful care. She was hospitalized for 10 days, and her arm

swelled to three times its normal size. They think she contracted this rare disease from a mosquito bite. Sometimes there were 7 to 8 doctors around her bed, because this is a disease which usually kills within 12 hours.

My mom was an avid walker, also doing water aerobics on a regular basis. I will never forget what one of the doctors said one day to my mom: "You would have died if your heart was not so strong. This kind of infection kills most people."

The time to get fit is not when you are sick. The time to get fit is now. When you are already sick, it is too late.

"I don't have time" can no longer be an obstacle to fitness. You *can* control your time. You have too much at stake, and you have so much to live for!

Obstacle #2: Boredom

I must admit, sometimes exercise can be boring. Many of my friends run on a treadmill day after day. Just the thought of that makes me want to quit! Boredom may be an obstacle you need to get over as well.

I went to visit a friend who was feeling discouraged about her workout commitment. Once again, she was lamenting her failure to stick to her exercise plan. Her goal was to walk on her treadmill fives times a week. I asked her to show me the treadmill. It was downstairs in a closed-off room with no windows and very bad lighting, and the machine was facing the wall. The problem was not her level of commitment—I sensed a strong desire in her to continue to exercise—the problem was the location of the treadmill! I told her to sell the treadmill and get outside and take a walk, even just a 10-minute walk, two times every day. With her personality, she was much more likely to take a walk to visit a friend than she was to lock herself away in the basement.

It is no wonder that she did not keep her commitment to get on that treadmill. Her exercise time seemed like time in a prison cell! Total isolation with no stimulation! What is boring to you may not be the exercise itself but the logistics of it. Set yourself up for success by honestly taking a good look at why what you're doing is boring. There are some people who love to spend 30 minutes on a treadmill without any distractions, but others need to watch TV while using the machine!

Another helpful tool to use is your imagination. I want you to think back and remember what it was like when you were a child. For most of us, childhood was not boring. We spent a great deal of time outside, playing and exploring the world around us. My mom would lock the door and tell us to stay outside and play until supper. Thinking back to those days, I remember being an active child. I ran or skipped more than I walked. I rode my bike every day (it was my absolute favorite toy). I jumped rope with the girls in the neighborhood. My sister and I climbed every tree in the neighborhood. And of course we played Hide-and-Seek in the summer until dark.

What did you like to do when you were a child? What kind of neighborhood did you grow up in? Were you in the country or city? Did you enjoy the water? Did you like to play games with others? Did you like to ride your bike by yourself or with a group of friends? Did you enjoy being outside? You may not be able to do all of the things you could do as a child, but you can recapture the spirit of how active you were. Don't forget how much fun it is to play! Exercise can be boring, but playing is fun!

Since I tend to get bored with almost anything pretty easily, I have to be creative in my exercise time. I love to cross-train, which simply means I work out in a variety of ways. On different days I walk, ride my bike, climb the rocks on the beach, and teach classes. On my walking days, I use the time as an extension of my quiet time and pray as I walk. On some of those days, I bring my favorite music and sing praises to God!

Here are some suggestions to overcome exercise boredom:

- *Play every day!* Make a list of five simple physical activities you enjoyed as a child. You may have to improvise or adapt some activities, but you can still enjoy them. Engage in one of those five things at least once a week. For example, as a child, my sisters and I loved washing our family station wagon. It was a chance to play in the water and do our chores at the same time.

• *Learn something new!* I remember the first time I tried Nintendo Wii. I thought it was going to be so dumb! I actually enjoyed it and worked out for an hour before I realized how much time I had spent using it.

•*Find a playmate!* Look for someone who you can share doing something fun with! After I finished the first draft of this book, I took a trip to Alaska for a week of kayaking and hiking with nine other women I had known for just a few weeks. The purpose of the trip was just fun—with a little bit of exercise for good measure. We worship a God who loves being creative, so take advantage of your God-given creativity, dig deep and discover ways to have fun and enjoy your exercise time. God has given you too many resources for boredom to be an obstacle. Enjoy the adventure of discovering great fun ways to stay fit.

Obstacle #3: No Visible Results

A typical conversation with someone who has given up on exercise might go like this:

Friend: I have been exercising, and it's not doing any good.
I have not lost any weight nor gotten any smaller.
Vicki: How long have you been doing this exercise routine?
Friend: At least two weeks.

Two weeks is not long enough. We cannot expect to undo years of neglect and lack of exercise in just two weeks. We did not get out of shape in two weeks, so therefore we cannot expect to get back in shape in two weeks. However, while it is absurd to think this way, when many of us don't see immediate results, we give up. One of my all-time favorite motivational heroes is Coach John Wooden. While at UCLA, Coach Wooden led his team to 10 NCAA national basketball championships in a 12-year period, so he obviously knew what brings results! He said, "Nothing works unless you do."

Consistency is the key to overcoming a lack of results, not the type of exercise you do, the time of day you exercise, what you eat before you exercise, what you drink when you are done exercising. None of those things matter—what matters is *perseverance*. In all of my years of teaching fitness, I have never found one person who, if consistent, did not get results from exercising. Consistent exercise will always pay off and bring results. Some results are easier to see than others, however, so it is important to set different kinds of goals. Using the scale to monitor your results can sometimes be discouraging. You can work really hard at eating well and exercising and the scale may barely move. It might seem as if all your hard work is not bringing any results.

This is exactly what happened with Wanda. She had been working hard at her wellness goals, but in eight weeks, she had only lost five pounds. I could tell she was thinking about quitting, or at least trying something different. But after a visit with her doctor, her whole attitude changed. Her blood tests revealed something remarkable: Her bad cholesterol had dropped 20 points in just eight weeks! She learned that with this kind of progress, it was entirely possible that she could come off of her cholesterol medications in just a few more months. Setting different kinds of goals will help you see different kinds of results.

I was so blessed by an elderly lady in my Body & Soul Fitness class. Janie suffers from osteoarthritis, which makes it painful for her to get down on the exercise mat. I encouraged her to keep trying, figuring that as she got stronger, she would be able to do more. Just this week, she told me that she had almost quit because exercising had been so painful, and for a long time she wasn't sure it was really helping. But she smiled as she told me, "This exercise class is helping my marriage!" Her husband has a boat and enjoys going out on the water, but she had never had the strength or enough flexibility to get in and out of the boat. This past week they took the boat down the river for an anniversary getaway, and she was able to get in and out of it by herself! She enjoyed every minute of the trip! And her husband was thrilled.

Janie and I learned what Paul told the Galatians to do when he was concerned they were giving up too quickly. Paul wrote, "Let us not become weary in doing good, for at the proper time we will reap a harvest if we do not give up" (Gal. 6:9). Imagine the harvest you'll experience if you remain consistent in your plan to get fit. Consistency will bring results—guaranteed.

Obstacle #4: Injury

Most of us start off really ambitious and just flat out overdo it. We don't take the proper precautions before we start exercising, and we don't give our bodies enough time to make adjustments.

Every year I witness this on the ball field. Since my four children have all been athletes, I have spent half of my life on a bleacher somewhere in South Carolina. The coed softball teams get together and play, and I never fail to see some guy come straight from work, change his clothes in the car, immediately step up to the plate, hit one deep into center field and burst out of the box, running full blast for first base. But because he didn't take the time to stretch, by the time he gets there he is limping like crazy because he pulled a hamstring. I can see it coming every time. You might have been able to get away with doing such a thing when you were 12 but not when you are 40, especially not when you consider that the last time you ran any distance at all was during last year's softball season!

Just so you don't think I sit in judgment of 40-year-old men, I have done the same thing myself. Just this past winter, I had some surgery that required me to rest for six weeks. On week seven—you guessed it—I started right back into jogging and overdid it. I hurt my back! By not taking my own advice, I injured myself and had to slow things way down. I had actually put myself at risk for complications from my surgery.

It is not as important to exercise hard as it is to *exercise smart*. Some ideas that we teach and practice at First Place 4 Health will help you stay safe as you start the exercise portion of your journey toward wellness:

- *Start smart.* Begin with just 10 minutes of exercise a day, twice a day. Increase the time slowly.
- *Start stable.* Support your feet to avoid injury. Foot pain is a common problem for beginners just starting to exercise, especially for those who have a lot of weight to lose. Extra cushioning insoles in your workout shoes will help with stability, impact and weight distribution.
- *Listen to your body.* When you get to the point of exhaustion, you have done too much. Exercise is supposed to be hard work, but you should not feel totally wiped out. You should feel tired but with a sense of wellbeing.
- *Learn to tell the difference between soreness and an injury.* Any muscle that has not been used in a while will feel sore after you exercise. The soreness should lessen after 48 hours. An injury is quite different. If unsure about an injury, it is always wise to consult your doctor.
- *Stay hydrated.* Water will give energy to hardworking muscle groups and will replenish the body fluids depleted from sweating.
- *Compete with yourself and no one else.* Alternate increasing time one day and increasing distance or intensity the next day.
- *Avoid the "too's": too much, too soon, too fast.*
- *Never, ever skip the stretch.*

You *Can* Do It!

Each of the top four obstacles to exercising *can* be overcome. But ultimately, you are going to be the one to determine how you will react when you're confronted by one or more of them. Although 80 percent of all people fail to continue their exercise program, you *can* be part of the elite 20-percent group who rises above. You *can* do it!

Developing an intentional plan to be above average in your wellness endeavors and putting forth the effort *to do it* will ensure success on your part. You will no longer be one of those people who quit after just a few weeks. You will be successful for the rest of your life.

As Coach John Wooden once said, "Success is peace of mind which is a direct result of self-satisfaction in knowing you made the effort to become the best of which you are capable." You do your part and God will do His part—and you will win!

Motivation for a Lifetime

Motivation matters. With the right motivation, things become possible. But what motivates us?

A young mom wants to get up early and have her quiet time with the Lord, but she just can't seem to get motivated. Suddenly, her young daughter is diagnosed with a rare but treatable cancer. The treatment is scheduled for 6:00 AM three times a week at the hospital. She no longer complains about getting up early. In fact, the mom goes to bed earlier than usual so she has the energy to get her daughter where she needs to go, and she even has time to take a shower and time for prayer. What was once "impossible" suddenly becomes doable. What's changed? Her focus.

What would motivate you to want to experience God's best for a lifetime? I want you to start thinking and praying about a motivation that will sustain you for the rest of your life—a motivation that will keep you following through with wellness commitments, even when things start to become very hard.

I love Proverbs 16:2: "People may think all their ways are pure, but motives are weighed by the LORD" (*TNIV*). We sometimes have a hard time understanding our own motivations because we tend to think we always have our own best interests at heart. But in reality, we don't. We can easily fool ourselves into thinking we have long-term goals to get fit, but at some point we quit and fail to reach those goals.

How many times have you convinced yourself that this time you'll stick to your commitment to get healthy, only to stop after some initial success? After three solid months of eating better and exercising, you begin to slack off, because you've lost 10 pounds and feel great. After all, you've already lost more weight than you expected and you feel better, so why not have that second helping of fries? You deserve it after all your hard work! Within weeks, however, the weight is back as well as that old familiar feeling of failure. *If I only had more willpower, things would be better,* you say to yourself. But willpower is not something you *find;* it's a direct result of your internal motivation. When you pray and submit yourself to the Lord, He helps you to "weigh" your motives and begins to make possible what seemed to be impossible: wellness for a lifetime.

Whether you are getting married, joining a Bible study, starting a new job or getting fit, what motivates you will determine how long you stick with your new commitment. In fact, if you tell me your motivation for getting in shape, I'll be able to predict just how long you'll stick with your commitment to stay in shape. I've seen it over and over again. So let me ask you: Why do you want to get fit? Be honest. The only wrong answer is a dishonest one. The more honest you are with yourself and God, the greater success you'll have in staying on track. So, why do you want to get fit?

As you consider this question, remember that there is a difference between short-term motivations and long-term motivations. Sometimes you might choose to get in shape for an event or a significant moment in your life, while at other times you might be motivated by more personal reasons. We will look at each of these in turn.

Motivated for a Big Event

When Jennifer told me about her daughter's upcoming wedding, she radiated excitement. Her joy, however, quickly turned to dread when she told me how she felt about appearing in the wedding photos. She needed to lose weight fast! I am always willing to help and encourage my friends, so we quickly worked out a diet, exercise and Bible-study plan to help her reach her goal. The day of the wedding, Jennifer looked great! She met her goal with hard work and determination. Honestly, I was so proud of her. When someone's motivated, anything is possible—with God's help.

That first week after the wedding, I was not surprised that Jennifer did not make it to our exercise class. Weddings take a lot out of a person. But when I still didn't see her after the second and then the third week, I began to wonder if everything was okay. Six weeks later, I ran into her at the grocery store, and you can imagine my surprise to see that she had gained back all the weight! Her motivation to look good for the wedding lasted just up to that final photograph at the reception. After the wedding, Jennifer no longer had the motivation to sustain her wellness disciplines.

Without a motive for the long haul, you won't keep your commitments, no matter how much you tell yourself, *This time will be different.* This is not to say that short-term motivations to get fit for a significant event in your life are bad or wrong. Feeling good about how you look for a honeymoon, family photographs, a family vacation or a high school reunion is a worthy goal. Why not look your best?

But here's the problem: A short-term goal will keep you on the roller coaster of weight loss. It is, after all, *short term.*

Motivated by Self-love

King David loved to write poetry. In reflecting on God's goodness, he wrote, "I praise you because I am fearfully and wonderfully made; your works are wonderful, I know that full well" (Ps. 139:14).

David described what is true about everyone and everything—God places a high value on each of His creations, including you. To acknowledge God's amazing work in creating you is not an act of self-focused egotism but rather an act of praise. The old bumper sticker is true: "God Don't Make No Junk." In order to have a healthy biblical perspective on your motives for healthy living, you need to place a high value on God's work in creating you. It is important to realize and appreciate your uniqueness. There is no one else exactly like you! You are God's special and precious child, and for you to appreciate what God has given you is simply another way to glorify God.

However, there is a danger to be aware of: Self-love may rear its ugly head when your healthy God-given joy becomes a self-focused, self-centered obsession with yourself—when *you* become the main focus of all your endeavors.

Being motivated by self-love might work well for a while—working out to look sexy or attractive compels many people to get into shape. You enjoy the way you look, so you work out. There's nothing wrong with enjoying who God has made you to be. But if your motive is only self-love, you will face one of two negative outcomes: self-obsession or self-neglect.

Danger of Self-obsession

Do you know anyone who has a meltdown if he or she doesn't get five miles of jogging in every day? How about someone who would not let a single serving of junk food pass through his or her holier-than-thou lips? When our motive to stay in shape becomes an obsession, we've crossed the line from living God's plan for our wellness to living our plan for ourselves. Our extreme attitude toward health no longer has a place for God, and we shut Him out from our lives. Instead, our endeavors become our god, and we engage in the practice of self-worship without even realizing it. Unfortunately, self-worship (in terms of health) has become a phenomenon in our culture, and self-care has morphed into self-righteousness.

In her article "A Feast Fit for the King: Returning the Growing Fields and Kitchen Table to God," Leslie Leyland Fields writes the following:

> To claim that certain foods lead through the narrow gate to purity and righteousness, and others lead down the wide road to pollution, is nothing new. A popular Hindi website, Food for Life Global ("Uniting the World Through Pure Food"), explains that only "pure vegetarianism" is allowed because what we eat directly affects "our spiritual consciousness" and our "subsequent behaviors." The very purpose of food, it says, "is to give strength to the body and purify the mind." Some strands of Buddhism also require vegetarianism. A woman writes on a food blog, "My desire to be a vegetarian is very tied up to my desire to be a Really Good Person." . . .

Strangely, while these writers offer a global, moral, even theological perspective on food, in practice their approach can lead to myopic self-absorption and legalism. In online social networks, people dish the details of their every meal and bite as if the world hung upon their words and their food choices. Some show signs of orthorexia, an eating disorder defined as "an unhealthy obsession with healthy eating." Colorado nutritionist Steven Bratman coined the term after his own journey into obsessively healthy eating while living on a commune and managing an organic farm. In his desire "to eat pure food," he rejected any vegetable plucked from the garden more than 15 minutes previously. For the sake of mindfulness, he ate alone and chewed each bite 50 times, all of which left him feeling "clear-headed, strong, and self-righteous." He writes, "A day filled with sprouts, umeboshi plums, and amaranth biscuits comes to feel as holy as one spent serving the poor and homeless."

Bratman's goal of achieving "wellness through healthy eating," though, began to take over his life. "I had been seduced by righteous eating. The problem of my life's meaning had been transferred inexorably to food, and I could not reclaim it." Today, Bratman, now restored, sees growing numbers of patients in his clinic with this disorder.[1]

The problem with self-obsession is that we simply cannot maintain these attitudes and keep a healthy view of the whole of our lives. We were not created by God simply to eat all the right foods and focus purely on that aspect of life. When our eating habits and exercise become all about us, then food and exercise have taken our eyes off of the Lord. We can become more concerned with our tight abs than with our quiet time with God. That may work for a while—maybe even years—but eventually the focus on self can ruin our view of ourselves and of God.

Suddenly, when we don't eat right or don't exercise, we think we have "sinned." Haven't you heard at least one person say, "I've been really bad this week—I had too much dessert." God loves us whether we eat dessert or not. We are not meant to obsess over what we do; rather, we are to be concerned with how we glorify God in what we do. We need to be careful, however, that we don't throw the exercise machine out with the bathwater and practice self-neglect.

Danger of Self-neglect

Evangelical Christians are one of the unhealthiest people groups. We love our church potlucks and Sunday afternoon brunches! Unfortunately, overeating is a part of our culture that we've embraced without thought or reflection. Instead of being in the world and not of the world, we are in it and loving it.

According to the most current statistics from the Centers for Disease Control, obesity is now considered an epidemic. It is a *conservative* estimate that approximately one-third of the population is obese.[2] That's inside the Church and outside the Church. Around one-third of those who consider themselves Christian are obese! How can this be? Are we truly practicing the Lordship of Christ if He is not Lord of our appetites and our activities?

> Do you not know that your body is a temple of the Holy Spirit, who is in you, whom you have received from God? You are not your own; you were bought at a price. Therefore honor God with your body (1 Cor. 6:19-20).

This verse speaks directly about taking care of our bodies. While Paul was specifically writing here about watching over our sexual activities, I wonder why we don't extend this verse to include caring for every aspect of our bodies. We'll sit with church friends and talk about the downfall of sexual mores while we enjoy our second helping of fried chicken and mashed potatoes. But God calls us to take care of our bodies—inside and out—in all areas of our lives. What we put into our bodies and how we stay in shape *do* matter to God.

Balance Between Self-obsession and Self-neglect

Our goal is to find a balance between self-worship—becoming totally obsessed with our health—and total neglect of our health. The

Bible clearly says that we are to have no other gods before Him (see Exod. 20:3; Deut. 5:7), and in Romans 12:3, Paul tells us, "Don't think more highly of yourself that you ought, but rather think of yourself with sober judgment, in accordance with the measure of faith God has given you." Somewhere between self-obsession and self-neglect we are to live and walk in truth.

One thing that can help us more than anything is our focus. If we can find a focus that has eternal value, we can avoid the pitfalls of the extremes mentioned above. I love what Paul writes in 2 Corinthians 4:18: *"So we fix our eyes not on what is seen, but on what is unseen. For what is seen is temporary, but what is unseen is eternal."* That means *I may have to focus on something that I cannot even see or may never get to see until I get to heaven.*

God has made you unique and wants you to enjoy and care for the body He's given you, but you were not simply created for you. While it *is* about you, it *is not all* about you. God wants you to be healthy and well so that He can use you in ways you cannot even imagine. You simply need to take the first step and look beyond yourself.

The Greatest Motivations

How do we take the first step? How do we look beyond ourselves? How do we discover the motivation that will last a lifetime? Actually, we don't need to figure it out, because Jesus has already told us.

One day, a religious leader confronted Jesus with a test. (Rabbis would often challenge each other to better understand God's Word.) In this particular test, the religious leader asked Jesus, "Of all the commandments, which is the greatest?" (see Matt. 22:35; Mark 12:28). The religious leader was hoping Jesus would pick one and then have something to argue with Him about. Jesus' response not only stopped this religious leader in his tracks, but also set the standard by which we all can "weigh" our motivations for everything we do:

> Jesus replied, "Love the Lord your God with all your heart and with all your soul and with all your mind. This is the first and greatest commandment. And the second is like it: 'Love your neighbor as yourself.' All the Law and the Prophets

hang on these two commandments" (Matt. 22:37-40; see also Mark 12:29-31).

Love God and love others. These are the two powerful motivations that help us avoid the dangers of self-obsession and self-neglect. Let's take some time to explore each of these two powerful motivations.

Motivated by Love for Others

Love for someone else—now that will get you moving! Let me tell you about my friend Cathy. Cathy is a widow living in Canada. She was a pastor's wife for many years until the sudden death of her husband. Now she is raising her daughter by herself.

Initially there were a lot of difficult adjustments, but they are making it. One of the hardest things Cathy had to deal with was her daughter's fear that she would lose her mom and be left alone. Cathy came to me and asked if I could help her get in great shape, because she wanted to help relieve her daughter's fear. Cathy is now doing the work she needs to do to achieve wellness, and I am sure she will be successful. Her love for her daughter is deeper and stronger than her love for herself, and that love has eternal value. Cathy is motivated for a lifetime.

Another friend of mine, Kay, came into my First Place 4 Health class and actually looked great for her age (she is in her mid-60s). When I asked her why she was joining our class, she told me that her oldest child had just had her first baby and she wanted to be there when her granddaughter, Emily, graduated from high school. "I want to be there when she gets married, and I'm not healthy. I may not be overweight, but I am not a healthy person." When it comes to exercise and eating, Kay's love for Emily compels her to make great choices every day.

One of the most influential Christians I know is Carol Kent. I met with Carol a few years ago when she asked me to help her develop a fitness plan. (You'll learn more about this plan in chapter 13.) Carol is a strong and mature Christian, but she realized that she needed to get healthy and stay healthy. When I asked her to share with me what being healthy meant to her, Carol told me that her only child, JP, is incarcerated in a federal prison in Florida. He murdered the father of his two stepdaughters after he learned that they were being harmed by the man. Sentenced to life in prison, he has no chance of parole—not ever.

Carol visits with her son almost every Sunday and is committed to caring for him and supporting him for the rest of her life. She feels that she needs to live a long, long time to be there for JP. Her motivation is sustainable because her motivation is her great love for her son. The time she has with him has eternal value and eternal benefits. Her encouragement in JP's life and in the lives of many others has benefits that go beyond this life into the next.

Let me introduce you to Kim Frketic. Kim's testimony touched my heart, and I hope it encourages you to think about how love for others might be the sustaining motivation you need to get fit for a lifetime:

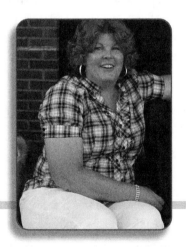 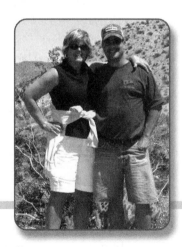

KIM FRKETIC

The turning point for me came a few years ago when I got on the scale and saw that my weight had crept over the 200-pound mark. My blood pressure was also dangerously out of control. I had all of the "head" knowledge from years of reading nutritional and weight-loss books, but somehow I had gotten off the right path and had no motivation to use all that knowledge.

Then along came Rayleigh Jo Nelson, my first precious granddaughter. Thinking about what life will be like watching her grow up, I realized that I would be an out-of-shape granny unable to keep up. It was time for a heart change. Over the past two years I have lost 25 pounds and reduced my cholesterol levels and my use of blood pressure medicine. Recently I have hit a plateau in my weight loss. It has been a good time to reflect and regain my focus and motivation and decide to press on and lose that next 30 pounds. I can really feel it when I climb hills. I am still on some medication, but I believe that one day soon I will be able to eliminate all medications.

For me the key is to be aware daily of what I put into my mouth. I keep a journal of the food I eat, and I focus on eating living and raw foods and lean proteins. I have to move every day! I used to believe that exercising a few times a week was enough, but as I get older, my body needs to move more. I love my bike and feel fortunate to live in a small town where I can ride my bike anywhere I need to go. I put a seat on the back for my granddaughter and away we go!

Besides the physical changes in my body, I have experienced spiritual changes as well. My heavenly Father has taught me so much on my wellness journey. Just today as I was following my husband up a steep and rocky hill, I became winded and my knee was aching. I was tempted to quit, but I knew the beautiful waterfall at the end would be worth the climb. I heard the Lord's voice saying, "This hike is a part of your journey: It's a long weary climb, but it's all worth it. Look what is coming ahead!"

I am thankful for my husband's encouragement, which keeps me moving, and for my sister, Vicki, who has been my mentor. Most of all I am thankful for my granddaughter, Rayleigh Jo. God has used her in my life for inspiration and motivation.

From the examples I've given, you can see that a person motivated by love for others can get moving along the road to wellness. These people really "get it," but "getting it" sometimes takes time. I think of another grandmother I know who is extremely obese and does not take care of herself. She has a precious little grandson who thinks the world of her. I have begged her to do something about her weight, but her response has always been, "I just can't do it." I don't know what it will take to get her to wake up and see what is at stake and how much she (and the ones who love her) have to lose if she doesn't take care of herself.

I also think about my own motivation. There was a time when I really just wanted to look cute. Again, there is nothing wrong with wanting to look cute, even though it's kind of shallow. A few years ago my oldest son headed off to the mission field, to a country that is not friendly, so to speak. He has planted his life in a country that is hostile to Christians. God has called him to a faraway, rugged place, and if I want to be a part of his life, I need to be fit enough to make the journey to see him where he is. I have a feeling he will meet his wife there; and my grandchildren will be born and live there too. I have a lot to live for and a lot to look forward to. I don't want to miss it because I can't stand up under the pressure of international travel and being subjected to an uncomfortably rugged lifestyle.

Love for others is a motivation that can last a long time and has eternal value.

Motivated by Love for God

Most people are motivated by the fear of losing something or the reward of gaining something. A smaller percentage of people are motivated by the simple fact that leading a healthy lifestyle is the right thing to do. That's really what love for our heavenly Father is—an act of obedience and love. It is love when we do the right thing for God because doing the right thing is pleasing to God (see Rom. 12:1). His love for me sustained Him all the way to the cross. I want my love for Him to sustain me as I take care of myself for as long as He leaves me here. That is truly where I want my relationship with God to be in my wellness endeavors.

There is so much to do for the Kingdom. God is at work in our world, and I want to be strong enough to join Him. He has called me to teach fitness, and if I become lazy, unhealthy or overweight, I will not be able to do this. God is using me and my wellness endeavors to bring people into His kingdom. He is using me to influence others, just as He will use you.

I have decided that I want to invest my time and energy in living a healthy lifestyle for one simple reason: It's a small investment with a huge return.

In many of His parables, Jesus taught that great things can come from small beginnings. As early as the fourth century, it has been suggested that the parables were told by Jesus to encourage His disciples to build the kingdom of God. I want to spend my time, energy and resources in building into the lives of people and into the kingdom of God.

The parable with the most impact for me regarding kingdom growth is the parable of the mustard seed, found in Matthew 13:31-32. The parable reads as follows:

> The kingdom of heaven is like a mustard seed, which a man took and planted in his field. Though it is the smallest of all your seeds, yet when it grows, it is the largest of garden plants and becomes a tree, so that the birds of the air come and perch in its branches (see also Mark 4:30-32; Luke 13:18-19).

In the parable, Jesus spoke of how the birds come and nest in the branches of the tree that grows from that smallest of seeds, which means that God's kingdom is destined for remarkable growth. That is part of what my purpose is about—creating a safe haven for people in need of health and weight loss and, at the same time, providing good news—the gospel of Jesus Christ—as they perch! As I continue to look to Jesus as Lord of my life, lives are being changed one pound at a time, one day at a time. These are some of the wonderful things that have happened as I have continued to love God and allowed Him to use me in helping people get healthy:

- My marriage was healed.
- I forgave my parents of child abuse.
- I learned to love myself.
- I sought God's forgiveness.
- I came to Christ.

- I got my life back.
- I became an athlete.
- God gave me the willpower to eat in moderation.
- I can feel God working on me and in my life almost every minute I live.
- I no longer carry around the burdens of guilt, anger and frustration.
- My days are filled with thoughts of Him, and I sing praises deep from within me, for He rescued me from my own miry pit.

Here is the story of my friend Molly, told in her own words:

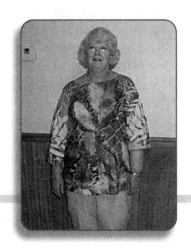 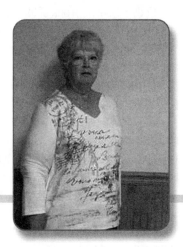

MOLLY DANIELS

When my second husband died suddenly, after we had been happily married for only eight years, I thought that at age 55, my life was over too. Tom and I had done everything together, and I'm afraid that he had spoiled me. I had not even put gas in the car in the entire time we were married.

Suddenly, I was left with the prospect of being responsible for myself. Tom had planned for me financially so that was no problem. I was eligible to retire from teaching, so I did just that. I tried to go to church, but it was just too upsetting. I got into a rut of not really caring about myself and stayed there for seven years. It was as though I was committing a slow suicide. I gained about 60 pounds, even though I am diabetic. I ate out frequently, socialized with just a very few friends and spent a lot of money to make myself "happy."

I don't know why, but having lived in the same small town my entire life, I was suddenly led to move away from everyone and everything I had known. I decided to move to Edisto Beach. I don't think my children thought I would really do it, but against all odds, I sold my house and found one I could afford at the beach. I promised myself that once I moved, I would take long walks on the beach and try to regain my health.

Needless to say, that did not happen the first year after I moved. I did return to church, joined several organizations and met many wonderful, caring people. It was as though I had to heal my emotional and spiritual being before I could start on the physical. Then out of the blue, I heard about an exercise class called Body & Soul from one of the first friends I met after moving to Edisto. She kept encouraging me to go and when a friend at church agreed to go with me, I knew the time was right to make a change. After the first class, I told my friend that I wanted to go only once a week so that I would not get tired of it. I also insisted on driving us to class so that it would be more difficult to renege on going each week.

I am now in the second session of Body & Soul Fitness and I have made some new friends. Even though I cannot yet do all of the exercises, I see improvement in my strength, stamina, balance and flexibility. I plan to participate for as long as the classes are offered!

Body & Soul is a program of acceptance, encouragement and friendship. Participants are not judged, and I credit that atmosphere with giving me the confidence to do something about my physical health and leading me further along my spiritual path.

Body & Soul has also led me to First Place 4 Health, which is helping me tremendously in both physical health and emotional and spiritual growth. I believe that it was God's plan to bring me to Edisto and revive my once-lost spirit.

I know of so many people just like Molly whose lives have been changed when their motivation was right. The kingdom of God is certainly a blessing to all who take refuge under its "branches." According to Matthew 11:28-29, Jesus said, "Come to me all you who are weary and burdened, and I will give you rest. Take my yoke upon you and learn from me, for I am gentle and humble in heart, and you will find rest for your souls." Jesus will provide rest and nourishment for our souls. He is the bread of life, He is the living water, and He can give us the encouragement and support we need to make changes that will glorify Him.

Jesus told His disciples that they would be a part of something that would grow and bless the whole world, and that needs to continue happening! I don't know about you, but I want to be a part of something big and powerful. I have told the Lord that I love Him with all of my heart, soul, mind and *strength*! That is why I do what I do. Finally, I have a motivation that will sustain me for my lifetime.

What about you? What is motivating you? It's time to take a long, hard look at why you might have quit in the past. What will be different this time? The deeper the love and the stronger the commitment, the more sustaining the motivation will be.

A New Way to Worship

I enjoy cooking. I love to discover new ways to create healthy, tasty and satisfying dishes. In fact, one of my greatest joys is watching our family enjoying a new meal together. It truly is a comfort to eat good food and connect with loved ones. What a wonderful way to share time together!

At First Place 4 Health, we encourage each other to enjoy the food we've been given. What I don't enjoy, however, is cleaning up. As a mom of four, I've done enough dishes to last a lifetime. You can imagine my surprise when I discovered that doing dishes could actually be an act of worship! I know it's hard to believe, but let me tell you about Brother Lawrence and the way he learned to practice God's presence in all that he did.

Before Brother Lawrence was Brother Lawrence, his name was Nicholas Herman. Herman joined the military and fought in the Thirty Years War in Europe. During this time he realized his deep need for God. He saw a tree in the winter that had no leaves and no fruit. The tree seemed dead but lived with the hope of spring. He realized that in many ways he too felt dead inside, and he longed for the life that God might give him.

When his time of service was through, Herman pursued God with his whole heart and joined a monastery. At that point he became known as Brother Lawrence. Not having enough education to become a priest, Lawrence served in the kitchen—cooking, serving and cleaning up after his superiors. While in the kitchen, he made a radical discovery: He could worship God as much in the kitchen as in the church. Seeing God's presence in the everyday things of life, he wrote:

The time of business does not with me differ from the
time of prayer; and in the noise and clatter of my kitchen,
while several persons are at the same time calling for different things, I possess God in as great tranquility as if I
were upon my knees at the Blessed Sacrament.[1]

Have you ever experienced trying to make dinner while several
people ask you for different things? If you are anything like me,
you wouldn't describe those times as times of "great tranquility."
But Brother Lawrence lived the second half of his life practicing
the presence of God. In other words, no matter where he was or
what he was doing, he was continually focusing on being aware
that God's grace was covering Him, that God's Spirit was with
him, and that he could give thanks for God's amazing love in Jesus. In other words, he *lived* a life of worship. In that worship, he
found great tranquility, and so can you. When you expand your
idea of what worship can be, you'll find both strength and peace
in the daily activities of life.

A Fresh Look at Worship

Most of us think of worship as something we do on Sunday morning with friends and family. We sit in chairs while the praise band
plays, or we sit in pews, admiring the beautiful stained-glassed
windows of the building. As we exit the church, our worship stops—
or does it? Many of us continue to worship but at a different kind
of altar. We head to the nearest all-you-can-eat buffet, giving praise
to God while we fill up our plates for a second and third time.
What if we could make a connection between our eating and exercise commitments and our worship?

I'll never forget the day when God impressed upon my mind
that how we eat and exercise can also be a way to glorify God. It
happened one morning when I was on a run. I wore an old T-shirt
that said "I never run alone" with a picture of a cross on it. I was
really struggling that morning, so I just started to pray. I gave
thanks for the strength I had to even put one foot in front of the

other; I prayed for my children; I prayed that God would help me make good food choices that day. By the time I looked at my watch, I had been jogging for 60 minutes! When I focused on the Lord, my body just kept going. My spirit and my body were blessed that morning. I decided that from that moment on, every opportunity I had to exercise would be a worship experience. Even when I am teaching a class, I take the time to mentally make a connection to God.

I love Jesus' invitation for us to be with Him in everything we do. In John 15:5, He said, "I am the vine; you are the branches. If a man remains in me and I in him, he will bear much fruit; apart from me you can do nothing." If we stay connected to Jesus in everything we do, then we'll bear much fruit. In fact, if we do things on our own, we won't produce any fruit that is of lasting value.

Since that "fruitful" run of prayer and praise, my exercise experiences have become about something more important than just me and my body. That dedicated exercise time has become a holy encounter with the living God. The same is true when I choose to deny myself unhealthy foods. I have discovered that God can satisfy me beyond my physical appetite. Presenting myself to Him daily, in this body He has given me, has become such a powerful part of my walk with Him, I can't imagine living life any other way. Remaining in and with Jesus consecrates my day and my efforts to become something holy, set apart to glorify Him and not myself.

Our Spiritual Act of Worship

As we discussed in the last chapter, motivation plays a big part in our ability to stick to our wellness commitments. As we grow closer to our heavenly Father, His presence in our lives will begin to have a life-altering effect on us. His love for us and our love for Him will become our reasons for wanting to obey Him, for wanting to place Him at the center of everything we do. Our whole lives can be a living sacrifice to God. Everything we do can be seen as an act of worship when we place God at the center, allowing Him to transform the ways we think and act.

The apostle Paul had a deep passion that everyone would understand that God's love is extended to all and that there is nothing we can do to cause God to love us more or love us less than He already does. In fact, Paul spent the final years of his life sharing that message of grace with everyone he met. In a letter written to the Christians in Rome, Paul spent the majority of the letter describing how God's grace, not our good works, invites us into and allows us to have a close relationship with God.

Then, in chapter 12 of his letter, Paul proclaimed an amazing truth: Because God loves us, we should, in turn, live lives that demonstrate God's love and mercy to others. Paul wrote, "Therefore, I urge you, brothers, in view of God's mercy, to offer your bodies as living sacrifices, holy and pleasing to God—this is your spiritual act of worship" (Rom. 12:1). In other words, we are to *live* a life of worship.

Let's take a good look at Paul's words in Romans 12:1 in order to gain a deeper understanding of what worship can look like.

"Therefore, I Urge You"
In the first 11 chapters of Romans, Paul explores sin, grace and Jesus' death on the cross. He speaks of how "in all things God works for the good of those who love him," and he tells us that we can "rejoice in our sufferings" (Rom. 8:28; 5:3). Some of the most well-known passages in Scripture come from these eleven chapters. The turning point occurs in chapter 12, when Paul moves from talking about concepts and ideas and begins to get practical. If this were a sermon, it would be the part where the pastor talks about how we can apply what we've heard to our own lives. That's why Paul begins chapter 12 with the word "therefore." Whenever you see a "therefore" in Scripture, you need to ask, "What's the 'therefore' there for?" In this case, Paul is pleading with us to pay attention to what comes next.

"In View of God's Mercy"
Paul summons us to action by drawing our attention to God's mercy and His compassion as demonstrated by Jesus' death on the cross. God has absolute love for us and the entire world and demonstrated it by coming to us in love when we didn't deserve it (election), by

cleansing us of our sins and giving us new life (regeneration), and by His desire that we go out and live a new and different life in the world, sharing His love with others (calling). Mercy is the key ingredient that allows you and me to remain in Christ. When you are having a bad day, take some time to consider all the mercies God has shown you throughout your life. Your bad day will be transformed into a day of gratitude, because you will remember how God's mercy overflows in the life of a believer.

"Offer Your Bodies"

Because God loves us completely and has done everything necessary for us to live with Him, Paul says that we are to present our bodies to God. According to the Old Testament, the Jews used to present animals as sacrifices to the Lord as a way of expressing their need for Him and their gratitude to Him. The word used for "sacrifice" by Paul in Romans 6:13—where he talks about not giving our bodies over to sin but instead presenting, or offering, them to God as a sacrifice—is a reference to that Jewish practice of sacrifice.

Most of us are comfortable with the idea of offering our spiritual lives to God. We hope that the Lord will help us cleanse our thoughts and our hearts. But we need to remember that our presentation of ourselves to God—our gift—also includes our bodies. Yes, our physical bodies.

Why would God even want our bodies? The Jews were supposed to bring the best of the best to the Lord, and let's be honest: There are times in our lives when our bodies are far from the best. But here's the amazing news: Just as our spirits are given new life in Christ, our bodies are also given new life. It's through us—including our bodies—that God does His amazing work. Our bodies and our spirits cannot be separated (at least not in this world).

In another letter, Paul wrote these often-forgotten words: "May God himself, the God of peace, sanctify you through and through. May your whole spirit, soul and *body* be kept blameless at the coming of our Lord Jesus Christ" (1 Thess. 5:23, emphasis added). The Lord sanctifies not just our minds and spirits, but also our bodies. Sanctification is the process by which we move closer and closer to Christ in this world. Gradually, as we make choices to conform our lives to God's ways, He works in us to help us become a clearer reflection of Christ. We present our bodies because God made us to live full and complete lives. If we allow our natural selves to rule our exercising and eating habits, we run the risk of not allowing God to do His greatest work of sanctification in us, because we've limited His options due to our health.

"As Living Sacrifices"

How are we supposed to present our bodies? "As living sacrifices." Up until the death of Jesus, God's plan included His people offering sacrifices regularly in the Temple. With Jesus, God did away with the need for regular sacrifices, but He did not do away with the idea of sacrifice. In effect, Paul says, "Now that we no longer need the old sacrifices, I want you to present your whole self as a living sacrifice. Christ has already done the work, making you acceptable in God's sight; now live out your life in such a way that others see God's love and glory through you."

Check out these powerful verses:

> Through Jesus, therefore, let us continually offer to God a sacrifice of praise—the fruit of lips that confess his name. And do not forget to do good and to share with others, for with such sacrifices God is pleased (Heb. 13:15-16).

Your life becomes the sacrifice. Imagine the power of your testimony if when someone asked you why you decided to eat healthy and get in shape, you responded, "God's given me a short time on earth, and I want to live as long and as productively as I can to show others His amazing love. So I need to be healthy to do that well." God will be glorified through you as a living sacrifice.

"Holy and Pleasing to God"

What does a living sacrifice look like? "Holy and pleasing to God." I think the word "holy" has gained a negative connotation in our culture. Nobody likes people who act "holier than thou." But Paul is not talking about that kind of holy. A sacrifice that was holy was a sacrifice that was perfect. It was the best sheep (or bull or ram) of the flock—no blemishes, no broken bones. That perfect animal would be set apart in order to be offered to God. Being "holy" means being set apart for God.

If you are to live your life as a living sacrifice, you must be holy, and the way to be holy is to live a life that is set apart from those things that would draw you away from loving God or from loving others. Holiness demands that we make a choice to be different.

But holiness, in the spiritual sense, can only come from Jesus. None of us is without blemish (or sin), so it's in Jesus that we find the ability to live as God wants us to live. He alone can make us holy. By turning to Jesus each day to ask for forgiveness and the power to live well, we are made holy. It's not our effort but His! He not only cleanses us but also gives us the power we need.

When someone asks me how I can maintain a lifestyle of Bible reading, prayer and exercise, I first tell him or her about Jesus, who makes it possible. It's not what I do but what He does through me. And the great part is that He can do that through you too. Literally, forgiveness and the choice to follow God's plan are what make your life acceptable, or pleasing, to God.

"This Is Your Spiritual Act of Worship"

When we live as a holy people set apart for God, our very lives become our worship! This is what Paul calls us to do: Live a life of worship. The Greek word for "worship" can also be translated as "service." In other words, our service to God is an act of worship. In contrast to the old sacrificial system of offering animals as worship, our lives become acts of worship when we present our bodies to God as living sacrifices. What I discovered that day on my run was that worship means everything. My hope is that when people see the way I love them and realize that I want them to be their best (body and spirit), they'll see my life as giving glory to God.

Our Lives as Living Sacrifices

There are many ways we can present our bodies as living sacrifices, holy and acceptable to God. One way, of course, is not to offer our bodies as instruments of unrighteousness but as instruments of righteousness. We've already talked about how exercise can be a form of worship. Let's consider how our food choices and even shopping can become acts of worship . . . yes, I said *shopping*.

As we have already discussed, the sacrifices that God found acceptable in the Old Testament were those animals that were free from blemishes and flaws. We are incapable of being such sacrifices on our own, so Christ made the ultimate sacrifice on our behalf. He is the perfect Lamb. What we can do, however, to present ourselves to God every day as a living sacrifice in our bodies is to keep them as pure as we can. We can also keep our bodies as healthy as we can by choosing the best foods for them and not filling them up with junk food that has no nutritional value. Such foods are not going to build up our bodies.

I would like you to consider that each time you make a sacrifice of what you should eat over what you want to eat, you are presenting your body as a living sacrifice—you are performing an act of worship.

Imagine you are out to dinner and are faced with a variety of healthy and unhealthy choices. You may choose to have a nice salad with the dressing on the side, and the act of placing the dressing on the side could remind you of what it means to be set apart. Ordering food and eating can become an act of worship!

Or imagine walking into the grocery store and shopping with the mindset of worship. As you begin to shop, you can thank God for the ability to choose and for providing all of the choices you have before you. Instead of heading to the processed foods in the center of the store, you decide to "shop the edges," choosing from fresh produce, dairy products and various meats. With each choice, you give God praise for the ways He has provided fresh food for you to enjoy. In this way, the acts of choosing food and of exercising can be presented to the Lord as sacrifices and become acts of worship! Now, these acts *will* cost you something, as they should. After all, most sacrifices don't come easy, but they do come with tremendous blessing.

The Cost of Sacrifice

I love the story in the Old Testament about King David and a man named Araunah. King David had brought a plague upon Israel and went to God seeking mercy. As the story relates:

> Then the angel of the LORD ordered Gad to tell David to go up and build an altar to the LORD on the threshing floor of Araunah the Jebusite. So David went up in obedience to the word that Gad had spoken in the name of the LORD.
>
> While Araunah was threshing wheat, he turned and saw the angel; his four sons who were with him hid themselves. Then David approached, and when Araunah looked and saw him, he left the threshing floor and bowed down before David with his face to the ground.
>
> David said to him, "Let me have the site of your threshing floor so I can build an altar to the LORD, that the plague on the people may be stopped. Sell it to me at the full price."
>
> Araunah said to David, "Take it! Let my lord the King do whatever pleases him. Look, I will give the oxen for the burnt offerings, the threshing sledges for the wood, and the wheat for the grain offering. I will give all this."
>
> But King David replied to Araunah, "No, I insist on paying the full price. I will not take for the LORD what is yours, or sacrifice a burnt offering that costs me nothing" (1 Chron. 21:18-24).

David knew the value of sacrifice that feels like sacrifice. Experiencing the temporary pain of sacrifice opens the door to experience the tremendous gratitude of blessing.

I would like you to consider every time you sacrifice sleep and get out of bed to meet with God as an act of worship. Every time you use the stairs instead of the elevator, every time you pick up your running shoes and turn off the TV, and every time you choose to engage your body in exercise—it is an act of worship and a costly sacrifice.

As a high school senior in Jacksonville, Florida, I was introduced to an organization called the Fellowship of Christian Athletes (FCA). We met monthly to hear an inspirational speaker and talk about the challenges of being a Christian athlete. Years later, I decided to help the FCA chapter at my kids' high school. In reviewing the organization's materials, I came across the most amazing creed. I started studying it and decided that it had some real merit. There are some ideas in this creed that we adult athletes who are pursuing wellness should consider embracing for ourselves:

> My body is the temple of Jesus Christ.
> I protect it from within and without.
> Nothing enters my body that does not honor the Living God.
> My sweat is an offering to my Master. My soreness is a sacrifice to my Savior.
>
> I give my all—all of the time.
> I do not give up. I do not give in. I do not give out.
> I am the Lord's warrior—a competitor by conviction and a disciple of determination.
> I am confident beyond reason because my confidence lies in Christ.
> The results of my efforts must result in His glory.[2]

Just let those words sink in for a minute. This is the ultimate motivation we have been looking for. This describes making our sacrifice out of love and devotion to the Savior. At the end of my boot-camp classes, we huddle up, say this prayer and then wipe our brows and hold out our sweat offerings for the Lord. We make the sacrifice, and then we pray that God will find our offerings acceptable and pleasing.

Start worshiping God in a new way. Make your body a living sacrifice, and "pay" what is necessary to make your offering acceptable and pleasing to God. The cost will be worth the payment.

The Importance of Rest

A few years ago, I had reached a plateau in my personal weight-loss goal. No matter what I tried, I seemed to be stuck. And then, like a gift from heaven, a wonderful opportunity came my way. At the time, I was teaching three exercise classes a week, and my life seemed balanced. Then I received a call asking if I would lead two early-morning classes. Both classes started at 6 AM, and I figured that the extra workouts would be just what I needed to move off my plateau and achieve my goals. But rather than losing weight, over the next six weeks I gained five pounds! What went wrong? How could I have exercised more and gained weight?

I lost sleep.

When I added the early-morning classes, I did not change anything else in my routine. I continued my late-night chores, and although I felt a little tired, I also felt very productive. The body will compensate for a lack of rest by craving more food. I did not realize that I was eating more during the day to help give me the energy I lacked because I was so tired.

All of our wellness endeavors will be for naught if we fail to follow a timeless, ancient command: Rest. Getting fit requires that we focus on two types of rest: (1) the amount and type of actual sleep we need each night to stay healthy, and (2) the relaxation of the mind and body and the recreation of the spirit, which we experience when we take time to pray and meditate on God's Word.

Let's face it: Most Americans are busy—overly busy. We've established a culture of busyness that is out of step with many other countries in the world. According to the International Labor Organization, "Americans work 137 more hours per year than Japanese workers, 260 more hours per year than British workers, and 499 more hours per year than French workers."[1] In addition to working longer hours, we also try to fit in multiple activities to keep ourselves and our children active throughout the week and weekend. We are overstressed and overworked! All this busyness takes away from a critical aspect of staying healthy—getting enough sleep. The lack of sleep literally sabotages our weight-loss and wellness commitments. In a study done at Kaiser Permanente Centre for Health and Research in Portland, Oregon, the researchers wanted to understand how sleep, watching television, stress, spending time on the computer, and depression impacted someone's ability to lose weight. Charles Elder, the lead author of the study, reported:

> When people are trying to lose weight, they should try to get the right amount of sleep and reduce their stress. . . . Some people may just need to cut back on their schedules and get to bed earlier. Others may find that exercise can reduce stress and help them sleep. For some people, mind/body techniques such as meditation also might be helpful.[2]

Rest and exercise can help unlock your body's ability to lose weight and stay fit. With our 24-hour society and open-around-the-clock stores, some of us have to literally make ourselves go to bed. The things that we feel need to be done will never be complete. There will always be one more load of laundry to fold, one more phone call to return, one more email to answer or one more social website to visit. Rest is neither an option nor a luxury: It actually is essential for maintaining good health, keeping a clear mind and maintaining a positive attitude. When you are tired, everything else in your life suffers.

A good night's sleep will actually work to help you stay committed to becoming a fit and healthy person.

An Age-old Problem

Lest we think that busyness is a problem from our century alone, read the words of King Solomon, who lived a fast-paced lifestyle of success and power. By the standards of any historical period, Solomon had it all. People came from all over the world, seeking out the king of Israel, wanting to enjoy his wisdom and the beautiful surroundings he had created for himself (and his many wives) in Jerusalem. But his success came at a cost, and toward the end of his life, he came to realize that cost:

> Unless the LORD builds the house, its builders labor in vain. Unless the LORD watches over the city, the watchman stands guard in vain. In vain you rise early and stay up late, toiling for food to eat—for he grants sleep to those he loves (Ps. 127:1-2).

What does the Lord grant to the ones He loves? Sleep. Sleep is literally God's gift to us. As we begin our journey of getting fit for a lifetime, we need to take advantage of all the gifts we've been given—and sleep needs to be at the top of the list.

A Good Night's Workout

Why is sleep a gift? The body does its best work while asleep. If we can establish strong and consistent sleep patterns, that time will give our bodies what they need to restore and rebuild themselves.

I had the wonderful opportunity to hear Dr. Richard Couey, a dedicated Christian and an expert in the field of nutrition (his book *Nutrition for God's Temple* is a must-read), lecture on what happens at the cellular level while we are asleep. He explained that when we are asleep, the cells in our body are hard at work. This work happens best not during our waking hours but when we are fast asleep. Most significantly, hormones are released during our time of rest. The release of the master hormone, melatonin, is definitely affected by our sleep patterns.

Melatonin is called the master hormone because it actually sets the pace for the release of all other hormones. It affects the release of dopamine, which is essential for cognitive thinking, and controls adrenaline, which affects our energy level for the next day. Increasing the secretion of the growth hormone is probably the biggest impact that the release of melatonin has on our bodies. The growth hormone rebuilds our bodies.

Sleep studies show that optimal sleep includes four stages, and it's during the REM sleep cycle that the growth hormone is released. You guessed it—a full eight hours of sleep is usually needed to reach the REM sleep. The growth hormone is a powerful anti-aging hormone, often called the youth hormone. But it also has a direct impact on our *body fat*.[3]

After you reach your maximum growth, which is approximately at 18 to 20 years of age, the body then uses the growth hormone to burn off excess glucose and reduce fat storage, especially around the waistline. As we age, the secretion of the growth hormone decreases. This is why when we're older, we can no longer eat anything we want without gaining weight like we could when we were young. (Remember those good old days?)

The growth hormone also works in partnership with the insulin our bodies produce. If we eat a huge meal at the end of the day, the body secretes insulin to balance the sugars instead of secreting the growth hormone. We want the growth hormone to be produced, not insulin. In other words, the "growth hormone won't come out to play when insulin is in the way." Our sleeping habits and eating habits work together, either to promote weight gain or weight loss.

Other benefits of the growth hormone include helping to maintain skin tone and elasticity, maintaining strong bones and muscles, stimulating repair of damaged tissue, improving mood and sex drive, and strengthening the immune system. All of these things working together can slow down the aging process. As we age, the growth hormone declines in the body, and thus aging accelerates as we continue to grow older. We grow older faster from 50 to 55 years old than from 45 to 50 years old. I don't know about you, but I really want the rest of my life to be the best of my life, and since I can help slow down the aging process by getting enough sleep, I plan to do just that. I laugh sometimes when I think about how much sleep I need. It's a lot of work to keep me looking young!

Research shows that seven and a half to eight hours of regular, consistent sleep are needed for peak performance (both mental and physical).[4] If you are not getting enough rest, you might exhibit some of the following physical symptoms (besides grouchiness):

- Headaches
- Lack of energy
- Nervous diarrhea
- Heart palpitations
- Overeating or not eating enough
- Depression
- Feelings of anxiety
- Difficulty concentrating
- Anger

I work hard at getting a good night's sleep. There are entire books written on how to get a good night's sleep, but some of my personal favorite sleep aids include the following:

- I exercise as early in the day as possible. Exercise raises the metabolism and may make it difficult to get to sleep if you exercise too late in the evening.
- I kiss all of my children good night. (Right now I have two at home and two in other parts of the world.)
- I have trouble taking in all the calcium I need, so I drink a glass of milk before bedtime.
- I read the psalms if I need to relax. They always give me a sense of God's nearness and peace.
- I make sure my bed smells great! Changing bed linens frequently and using a pillow spray also help me look forward to crawling into bed.

A Word About Stress

Stress—a state in which we experience greater pressure than usual, physically, mentally or emotionally—is something we all encounter. Phrases such as "stressed-out" or "I'm so stressed" reveal the negative way most people view stress. But there are many positive aspects of stress as well.

Benefits of Stress

In contrast to popular belief, some stress is beneficial. In fact, we need it. Stress can push us to accomplish more and can actually energize us (such as by enabling us to exercise). In the same way, we can look at the challenges life throws our way and embrace them and allow them to energize us instead of draining us of all our energies.

The amount of stress on our bodies and minds can act in a positive way, making us feel challenged, excited and motivated. However, when we move past the mental and physical limits of the amount of stress we can handle in a healthy manner and we become overwhelmed, we will experience unpleasant physical and emotional consequences. This is when stress becomes distress! While positive stress may help you excel, too much stress can actually kill you.

I have come to realize that I can control the amount of stress in my life by controlling the major contributor of stress in my life. The major contributor to overstressing ourselves is . . . us! Many of us seem to lack the ability to say no to doing anything that is asked of us. I believe the average American man or woman is in a state of constant stress overload. The majority of families in our culture today are overcommitted, parents and children alike. There was a time in the Heath household when we lived what I like to call "life in a blender." You put everyone in the blender—Mom, Dad and all four children—and then throw in a lot of school pressure and work and sports and church commitments. Then you put the lid on and turn it on full blast! That's the American way—living life at warp speed!

The Danger of Internalizing Pressures

Many of us internalize during times of stress, but bottling things up is one of the worst things we can do, as it causes a volatile buildup of negative emotions that may explode at anytime. How we react to stress is determined by our ability (or inability) to meet the many demands made on our time and energy. Pressures come from outside us—family, friends, jobs, school, church—but they also come from within.

Sometimes the pressures we create—the internal pressures—are the most significant, because we make standards for ourselves that are impossible to fulfill. This same phenomenon occurs when we continually strive for perfection—it increases the stress. Can you imagine the impact this kind of distress can have on the body over the course of a lifetime of living with overly high self-expectations? While stress is not actually a disease, it certainly has an impact on disease and illness!

The Response to Fight or Flight

Our bodies are created to survive and are finely tuned to make certain adaptations to assure that we *do* survive! When we come under a stressful situation, messages are sent through the body and certain chemicals are released—primarily adrenaline and cortisol. Adrenaline and cortisol prepare us mentally and physically for survival. These two chemicals are responsible for the "fight or flight" syndrome. When cortisol and adrenaline are released in our bloodstream, our bodies prepare to stay and fight whatever must be confronted or flee from the present danger. Three predictable physical reactions automatically happen in the body when this occurs:

1. The body's metabolism slows down to conserve excess energy for the fight. This explains the sometimes-quick weight gain that often accompanies unresolved stressful situations. When stress hits, adrenaline mobilizes fat (excess energy) from all over the body and then cortisol takes what is not used and stores it in the midsection of the body. Other side effects of the body's slowdown include gastrointestinal disorders such as constipation, ulcers, colitis and diarrhea.

2. Blood sugar drops during times of stress, which then stimulates the appetite to call for usually high-calorie foods needed for quick energy release.

3. When stressed, the body will retain excess fluids in order to keep our systems lubricated and hydrated for survival.[5]

These responses to stress literally kept our ancestors alive! And they still function today to keep us alive in dangerous situations. The problem for us comes when we do not get to experience the resolution of the stressful situation.

Results of Chronic Stress

Unresolved stress upsets the basic chemistry of our bodies all the way down to the cellular level. And, unfortunately, many of us live in a chronic state of stress. Recent research has linked reactions to chronic stress to the development of several illnesses:

- *High blood pressure, heart disease, stroke, and atherosclerosis (the narrowing of the arteries due to a buildup of cholesterol).* Many people experience a small change in blood pressure during stressful times, but when stress is chronic, high blood pressure can become very dangerous.

- *A weakening of the immune system.* Some of the chemicals released during stressful times can decrease the number of white blood cells in the bloodstream that fight off infection, making a person more susceptible to illnesses such as the common cold and flu.

- *Anxiety and depression.* There is a sense of wellbeing that is associated with the resolution of a stressful situation. When stress is not resolved, a person can become overwhelmed, which can lead to depression.[6]

Jesus, Busyness and You

Busyness and fatigue are killing the American family. Couples are too tired to have sex, too tired to raise children and too tired to pray. I once heard someone say, "We are trying to go at Mach speed in a camel's body. We are not designed to live life this way, to pursue such a fast-paced lifestyle." Living life at Mach speed is not what God intended for us. Let's take a look at how Jesus gently confronted a busy friend who had put her priorities in the wrong place. Jesus enjoyed spending time at the house of his friends Mary, Martha and Lazarus. He would often use their house as a place of retreat and refreshment and to teach His disciples about the abundant life the Lord had for them. The Gospel of Luke recounts a time when Jesus needed to confront Martha about her tendency to crowd out what was most important with the urgent concerns of the present. As you read this account, try to identify some of the characteristics of the overbooked life.

> As Jesus and his disciples were on their way, he came to a village where a woman named Martha opened her home to him. She had a sister called Mary, who sat at the Lord's feet listening to what he said. But Martha was distracted by all the preparations that had to be made. She came to him and asked, "Lord, don't you care that my sister has left me to do the work by myself? Tell her to help me!"
> "Martha, Martha," the Lord answered, "you are worried and upset about many things, but only one thing is needed. Mary has chosen what is better, and it will not be taken away from her" (Luke 10:38-42).

What can we learn from Martha, Mary and Jesus about an overbooked life? In her study *Living Beyond Yourself*, Beth Moore points out that overcommitted people suffer from the four *D*s: distraction, doubt, deserted and demanding.[7] Too much activity was distracting Martha in the same way that too much activity can distract us from the real purpose of life.

Did you notice what was distracting Martha? Serving Jesus! Her problem had to do with the way she was going about her relationship to Christ. Beth Moore tells us that "serving Christ will never substitute for intimacy with Christ."[8] Have you ever felt as if you were doing and doing for the Church or Christ and getting less and less satisfaction? If so, it might be time to reduce your activity and go back to intimacy.

In fact, intimacy with Christ will produce service in the form of an easy yoke and a light burden (see Matt. 11:28-30). Are you striving so hard that you cannot rest? If so, your life is overbooked.

Doubting God's Love

Notice how Martha addresses Jesus when she's busy doing all the work and Mary's busy doing all the listening. She asked Jesus, "Don't you care?" I often wonder if Mary and Martha had this discussion all the time. Martha was tired of telling Mary what to do, so she placed the blame on Jesus. After all, shouldn't He tell Mary to get up and grab the dishes for dinner? Martha's view of the situation was distorted. She saw Jesus as not caring, but in reality, He cared deeply and wanted Martha to see the answer to her own dilemma.

When we have a proper view of God, we do not blame God for not caring about our busy schedule (a busy schedule that *we chose* for ourselves), but seek God for answers in the midst of our busy schedule. First Peter 5:7 says it this way: "Cast all your anxiety on him because he cares for you."

Feeling Alone and Deserted

Martha complained that she was doing all the work, and her sister was not helping with any of it. I have noticed, at times, that I feel the same way. I find myself thinking, *Am I the only one at this church who can do anything?* Such moments of self-pity can easily become seasons of disillusionment if we don't take the time to get God's perspective.

Being Demanding

The assumption is that busyness is correct, so everyone else should fall into line. *Everyone should have to suffer like me!* Overcommitted people want you to get overcommitted with them. They want you to be too busy too. Jesus loved Martha and responded to her, "Martha, Martha." He knew she needed help, but it was not help in the kitchen.

Allowing Other Things to Crowd Out the Main Thing

None of the things Martha was doing were as important as what she needed to be doing. Resting and sitting down to listen to Jesus was what she most needed. I don't believe Jesus was saying that serving Him was not important. Rather, I believe He was saying that *being with Him empowers us.* What I think is the key is what He said to her at the end of their discussion, "Mary has chosen what is better."

Psalm 16:11 says, "You have made known to me the path of life; you will fill me with joy *in your presence,* with eternal pleasures at your right hand" (emphasis added). Once again we discover that true joy originates in the heart and the personality of God: "I have told you this so that my joy may be in you and that your joy may be complete" (John 15:11).

Sabbath—God's First Plan

When we over-commit our lives, we leave no space for spiritual wellness in our hearts. Under what conditions are our souls restored? When is the oil of gladness poured out on us? It is during times of solitude and stillness, what the ancients knew as the practice of Sabbath. Practicing Sabbath means more than just going to church on Sunday. Within the very fabric of creation, Sabbath has been woven into God's direction for us to live a healthy life. Sabbath is the practice of taking time to communicate, have fellowship, and rest with the God of the universe. We need to take time to be with God and with our families and rediscover (each week) refreshment of the soul.

I find it fascinating that when God designed the universe, He gave the man and the woman their job descriptions: to take care of the Garden and to be fruitful and multiply (sounds fun!). But once He had declared everything good and everything was in position to be fruitful, God said, "Take the day off." On the seventh day, He Himself rested, and all of creation was to follow His example. From that time on, setting aside a day to rest and to remember our relationship with God has been the best way to live a healthy lifestyle.

Why do so many Bible-believing Christians ignore this primary command? I wonder if in America we are more concerned with keeping up with the Joneses than we are in keeping in line with Jesus. Jesus was pretty clear: If we want a life of getting fit and staying fit, we need to stay connected to Him (see John 15:5-6).

Stay Connected

If Jesus were alive today, He might be considered the ultimate life coach. He literally spent three years with His followers, not only instructing them on how to live, but also living life in front of them as a model. His mission was to help everyone experience an abundant life (see John 10:10). In one of His teaching sessions with His disciples, He spoke this great nugget of truth:

> I am the vine; you are the branches. If a man remains in me and I in him, he will bear much fruit; apart from me you can do nothing. If anyone does not remain in me, he is like a branch that is thrown away and withers; such branches are picked up and thrown into the fire and burned (John 15:5-6).

What a powerful image! Grapes are connected to branches. Those branches are connected to vines. The vines have roots that go deep into the soil to collect the food and water needed to create plump and juicy grapes. If the branch becomes disconnected from the vine, it will eventually dry up—no grapes, just a dead branch that can be used for firewood (at best!).

If we want to live the abundant, juicy lives that God has for us, what do we need to do? Stay connected. In our culture of living "life in a blender," we can easily get distracted from staying connected, but if we get disconnected, we'll soon be feeling like the dried-up twig on the side of the road, wondering what happened to the blessed life.

Here's the problem: We often don't even notice that we have become disconnected. We've become so used to the feelings of stress, exhaustion and dryness that we've forgotten (or perhaps have never known) the joy we can experience every day when we live by following God's priorities instead of our own. Remember, Jesus said that when we stay connected to Him, we will bear much fruit.

Slow Down

Deciding to slow down is one of the hardest things I have ever done. It was so hard for me because I was afraid—afraid I would miss something, afraid I would be left out, afraid my kids would fall behind, afraid, afraid, afraid. But should my schedule really be dictated by fear? Absolutely not.

When our family finally started slowing down, we actually were able to live by faith. We finally were able to literally live out what we proclaimed as Christians that we believed. We believe that God will meet all of our needs. We believe that He is a good shepherd and will care for us and will love us. The fear that we as a family might be found lacking in something was actually preventing us from receiving God's wonderful pastoral care.

I rest in the powerful and familiar words of Psalm 23:1-3: "The LORD is my shepherd, I shall not be in want. He makes me lie down in green pastures, he leads me beside quiet waters, he restores my soul." What is stopping you from letting Him be your good shepherd, allowing Him to restore your soul with the oil of gladness?

Retreat

Perhaps we would feel our need for God more if we denied ourselves the constant distractions that fill our lives. Maybe we need to practice removing ourselves from the distractions, to go somewhere alone where we can meet and see Jesus in a new way. Lessening our communication with others might increase our communication with God.

A few years ago, I was part of a retreat where we were asked to participate in a 24-hour fast of silence. We were not to talk to anyone for one full day. We were instructed to use the silence to try to hear the voice of God speak to us. For some of us, the silence wasn't so bad. I talk for a living, so having a few hours to not have to think of anything to say was refreshing. I discovered, though, that it was extremely difficult for some. Some of the people at the retreat seemed afraid of the quiet. Some may have been addicted to noise. Talking and noise can be welcome distractions when we are not interested in hearing what God has to say.

What I discovered was that removing the noise that fills our lives puts us in a position to receive God's silent grace. This grace that God wants to bestow on us requires that we participate by being completely still. When we rush through life at warp speed, with the music of life playing full blast, we are bound to miss this grace.

God's silent grace has come to me in the quiet moments just before the dawn, when I choose to get up and experience the sunrise with Him. His silent grace comes in the love of my husband who reaches over, saying nothing, and places his hand on my head in the night. His silent grace comes to me in the embrace of my children when they first wake up and come to find me. They don't need to say anything; just crawling up in my lap says it all. And I believe that God's silent grace will come to you.

Rest in God's silent grace. Allow His gift of sleep to strengthen your body as you continue to pursue Him.

A New Relationship with Food

"Food, glorious food!" are words from the opening song from the musical *Oliver!* written by Lionel Bart. It's sung in the scene where the workhouse boys are fantasizing about food while getting their bowls of gruel from the cook staff at the workhouse. These boys are overworked and underfed, something to which most of us cannot even begin to relate. But we do the same thing the boys in the workhouse did: We fantasize about food, glorious food!

I hate to devote an entire chapter of this book to our relationship with food, but I have to do so. The sad truth is that we will not be successful in meeting our wellness goals through exercise alone. Most physicians agree that optimal health is achieved 30 percent by what we do and 70 percent by what we eat. In fact, trying to manage weight with exercise alone can give way to the dangerous habit of exercise bulimia—the act of purging the body of calories through over-exercising. For optimal health, we have to incorporate two disciplines into our lives: exercising *and* eating quality foods in proper quantities.

Our Obsession with Food

Many of us wake up with food being our first thought and go to bed with it being the last thing on our minds. In our American culture, food has become one of the major focuses of our lives. We are obsessed with the crunchy, salty, sweet, cool and creamy effects of food. What has happened to us? There was a time when food was considered fuel and sustenance for the family, not a hobby or an indulgence.

We in America are certainly obsessed with eating. When we are an hour late sitting down to a meal, how many of us say, "I am starving to death!" That is definitely not the case! We Americans, on average, overfeed our bodies by 30 percent. Americans are getting bigger and bigger and, sadly, believers are leading the way.

In a study performed at Purdue University, Professor Ken Ferraro found that God must certainly love the overweight because "he is cranking them out by the score, at least among his devoted worshipers in certain American Protestant denominations."[1] In the study, Ferraro wanted to find out if there was any significant relationship between religious behavior and an unhealthy body mass index. What he discovered was that those states with a larger population of people professing a religious affiliation had a higher-than-average number of overweight and obese people.

The study showed that 1 percent or less of those claiming the Jewish, Muslim, Hindu, Buddhist or some other non-Christian religion qualified as being obese. The obesity statistics increased significantly among Christians (especially fundamentalists): around 17 percent of Catholics, 18 percent of Methodists, 20 percent of Pentecostal and Assemblies of God parishioners, and 27 percent of the fundamentalists, including the Southern Baptist, North American Baptist and other fundamentalist sects, were considered obese.[2] Lord, have mercy and pass the potatoes! It looks like we are nourishing much more than our souls.

This does not come as a surprise to those of us raised in the Bible Belt (the southern part of the United States). For most of us, the Christian social culture involves fellowship gatherings featuring home-baked pies, fried chicken, potluck dinners, church picnics and ice cream socials. These are such a part of Southern culture that they have become a part of our religious DNA. We've lived with a huge blind side: We preach against overindulging in alcohol, tobacco and even the kind of media we watch, but gluttony seems to be one of the few "overindulgences" that we have decided to embrace.

Steve Reynolds, pastor of Capital Baptist in Annandale, Virginia, says in his book *Bod4God* that he was amazed that his church let him stay in the pulpit when he weighed more than 300 pounds. If he had been preaching heresy, he says they would have fired him. He was obviously controlled by the sin of gluttony, but they allowed him to preach week after week, and no one said a word.[3]

One explanation for the lower obesity rate among Jews, Muslims, Hindus and other non-Christian faiths is the dietary restrictions inherent in following the beliefs of those religions. The Christian faith, however, has no restrictions. Christian denominations have complete dietary freedom, and we are now paying the price. Yet even with this bleak picture, there is great hope for Christians. More and more pastors have embraced the "whole person" concept and preach total wellness from the pulpit. They are preaching a theology that says we need to be healthy in all areas of our lives—physically, emotionally and mentally, as well as spiritually.

We can no longer use food to "fill us up." As Solomon wrote, "All man's efforts are for his mouth, yet his appetite is never satisfied" (Eccles. 6:7). Continued trips to the refrigerator and snack cabinet are not meeting the deepest needs of our hearts. We are not going to find what we need for soul satisfaction in an all-you-can-eat buffet line. I have a magnet on my refrigerator that reads, "It's not in here." It's a great reminder that when I am absent-mindedly wandering toward the refrigerator when my soul is feeling restless, the food I need is not in there. God has the best food plan ever.

Jesus' View of Food

Jesus loved to eat. In fact, His enemies accused Him of being "a glutton and a drunkard" (Luke 7:34). He knew how to enjoy a feast and how to celebrate at weddings with His friends. I imagine that Jesus fully enjoyed and savored the wonderful foods of Israel. But Jesus also knew that food could never supply His ultimate need for soul satisfaction.

While Jesus traveled in the heat of the day through Samaria, He came to a well and decided to rest. His disciples headed into town to buy some food. While Jesus relaxed at the well, a woman from Samaria came to draw water. To make a very powerful scene short, she eventually became one of the first to sense that Jesus was the Christ.

When the Samaritan woman left to tell the village about her good news, the disciples came back with food and offered to give Jesus something to eat. I'm sure the disciples wanted to make sure Jesus kept up His strength and energy. Check out what happened:

> Meanwhile his disciples urged him, "Rabbi, eat something." But he said to them, "I have food to eat that you know nothing about." Then his disciples said to each other, "Could someone have brought him food?" "My food," said Jesus, "is to do the will of him who sent me and to finish his work" (John 4:31-34).

Jesus loved food, but He understood that ultimate satisfaction comes from living in God's will and doing His work on the earth. How often have you been bored and mindlessly munched on chips? When you are seeking to live God's will, you will rarely (if ever) get bored, because your ultimate satisfaction will come from helping others to see God's amazing love.

Emotional Responses to Food

God created us with the mysterious and complex ability to feel emotions. We know that our emotions are an innate part of who we are. The Bible is full of passages that demonstrate the legitimacy of the emotions we feel. For example, we are told to "rejoice with those who rejoice; mourn with those who mourn" (Rom. 12:15).

Even though the Scriptures confirm that our feelings are part of God's good and perfect design of us, we often label our emotions as either good or bad. Joy is good, and grief is bad. Happiness is good, and sadness is bad. Emotions, however, are neither good nor bad. Emotions are neutral and serve an important purpose in our lives. But what we do with our emotions—now that makes all the difference in the world.

Jesus and Emotions

Jesus was a very emotional man. We see many examples of this in the New Testament. He was, at various times, compassionate, zealous, angry, sorrowful, delighted, troubled, joyful, greatly distressed, and even depressed (see Matt. 26:37; Mark 3:5; 10:14; 14:33; Luke 7:13; 10:21; 12:50; 19:41; John 2:3,15-17; 11:35,38). As children of God, we have the freedom to demonstrate the same full range of emotions, just as Jesus did. Our challenge is to demonstrate them *in the appropriate manner* and *at the appropriate time* and *direct them toward the appropriate person or situation.*

Emotional Balance

We often connect emotions with food memories. For example, I have a fondness for pizza. One of my favorite memories is from a time when I was about four years old and my father worked as a cook at the Officers' Club.

Dad was enlisted in the Navy, and we were stationed in Norfolk, Virginia. He would work very late in the evenings, and my mom would sometimes let me and my sister stay up to wait for him to come home. Many nights he would bring home a homemade pepperoni pizza, and we would sit around the coffee table and eat it together. So you can imagine that when I am feeling a little lonely for my dad, who passed away two years ago, I can be tempted to use a pepperoni pizza to take care of that loneliness. I can tell you right now, a pizza does not take the place of my dad. In fact, when I overeat pizza, I only feel shame and guilt.

Here are three principles to remember when it comes to understanding our emotions:

1. *We were not created for our emotions; our emotions were created for us.* We were not created to be ruled by our emotions and to allow our emotions to dictate the amount of food we deny ourselves or put into our bodies. Instead, God gave us emotions so that we can identify our values and what is important to us. When we cry because someone we know is hurting, we are expressing

the value of that relationship. Our emotions were created to help us understand what is important in our lives.

2. *Emotions are a barometer of our soul.* Emotions allow us to identify when something doesn't line up with what we believe or think. Experiencing a strong negative emotion is an indicator that something isn't resting well in our hearts. The challenge is to use that emotion to explore what is wrong and to work with God to resolve the imbalance.

3. *We can have emotional control.* Even though we have a long history of "being controlled" by our emotions, emotional balance is still possible. Whether we manage or mismanage our emotions, as we take them to the Lord, He will help us develop self-control and learn to rely on the Holy Spirit to achieve the appropriate emotional responses to the situations we face.[4]

Being Christian does not guarantee a life free from disappointment and discouragement. The reality is that our lives are full of situations that may result in emotional pain or even trauma, so it is essential that we learn how to appropriately handle those feelings and emotions before we end up, as Steve Reynolds says in his testimony, "literally digging [our] grave with a knife, fork, and, of course, an ice cream spoon."[5]

Instead of responding to our emotions with food, we are called to give everything we experience to God: "Cast all your anxiety on him because he cares for you. Be self-controlled and alert. Your enemy the devil prowls around like a roaring lion looking for someone to devour" (1 Pet. 5:7-8). Satan is the great counterfeiter, because he knows he cannot compete with God. Jesus said that He was "the bread of life," and the strength we gain from feasting on His Word can get us through any trying situation (John 6:35,48). Satan, however, tries to convince us that

Little Debbie Cakes are the bread of life and that they are the best choice for getting us through trying situations. But snack cakes are cheap substitutes for the powerful and awesome and compassionate God who cares for us!

Scripture instructs us to give our burdens to God, instead of trying to make them go away with the temporary good feeling we associate with overeating. We simply need to let God take care of us!

Emotions, Food and You

If you find yourself running to the refrigerator more than you run to God, you might be using food to meet needs in your life that only God can meet. Take a moment to ask yourself these questions:

- Do I sometimes put food in my mouth before I realize I've done it?
- Does eating cause me to feel stressed or guilty?
- When I get in a disagreement with someone or I'm bored, do I think of eating?
- Do I eat more when I have a lot of time on my hands?
- Have I developed a strategy for dealing with my emotions that doesn't involve eating?
- Does eating something fattening early in the day negatively affect my food choices for the whole day?
- Do I consider food my enemy?
- Do I wander around thinking, *I want something to eat, but I don't know what it is. What do I feel like eating?*
- Do I crave something to eat, even when I'm not hungry?
- Do I sometimes snack to avoid doing something else I need to do?

If you answered yes to any of these questions, you might be using food as a way to deal with your emotions. I would strongly encourage you to pray right now and ask God to show you the relationship with food and your emotions. Ask the Holy Spirit to speak to you and give you direction for your next step.

Forming a New Relationship with Food

It's helpful to know that God intended food to be good for us, to be fuel for us and to even be a comfort to us. We can enjoy our food with great freedom and with God's blessings. It's wrong to think, *If it tastes good, it must not be good for me.* God has given us beautiful, colorful, good-tasting food with which to nourish our bodies. As the writer of Proverbs 24:13-14 states:

> Eat honey, my son, for it is good; honey from the comb is sweet to your taste. Know also that wisdom is sweet to your soul; if you find it, there is a future of hope for you, and your hope will not be cut off.

Just as wisdom to live is a gift from God that is good for the soul, so too food is to be enjoyed as a gift. Unfortunately, food becomes so much more than a gift to us. We often use it as a substitute for a closer relationship with God, family and friends.

Food Is *Not* Your Relationship with God

I need to warn you about two different reactions people often experience when they decide to incorporate their faith and their desire to get fit:

1. *A feeling of superiority:* When you practice good eating, you feel superior to others and you may even feel as if you are walking more closely with God.

2. *A feeling of inferiority:* When you fall away from your weight-loss goal, you feel totally inferior to others and you sense that the Lord is somewhat disappointed in your inability to keep moving toward your goals.

We need to be careful of "food righteousness." Food righteousness is believing that what you choose to put in your mouth is what determines your righteousness (or unrighteousness). In other words, if you choose good food, then you are righteous; if you choose bad food or more food than you actually need, you are unrighteous.

In Romans 14:17, Paul says, "For the kingdom of God is not a matter of eating and drinking, but of righteousness, peace and joy in the Holy Spirit." The folks in the Early Church had an interesting relationship with food. Because of dietary laws set out for the Jews and some of the pagan practices of eating food that had been offered in a sacrifice to a pagan god, the Early Church (which had some members who had been Jewish and some who had been pagans) associated some of the food they ate with their sense of being right with God. In writing to the church at Rome, Paul wanted to set the record straight: Food is a non-issue with the Lord. While Christians can make healthy or unhealthy choices about food, the food itself does not determine what they are or how they relate to God. Paul encouraged the early Christians by instructing them that neither what they ate nor what they drank would have any better or worse effect on their relationship with God. After all, what makes people right before God? Actually, the better question is *who* makes people right before God. God does. If we want to experience the blessing of being in God's kingdom, we need to experience the Holy Spirit, who brings righteousness, peace and joy when we believe in Jesus Christ.

I love how David used the language of food to describe his relationship with the Lord in Psalm 63:5: "My soul will be satisfied as with the richest foods; with singing lips my mouth will praise you." Our relationship with God is defined by worship, not dessert. If you want to experience peace and joy, put down the ice cream and ask the Lord to meet your deepest needs. Allow Him to be the Lord of your emotions. Don't accept any false substitutes when it comes to righteousness, peace and joy. Let your first thought of the day and your last thought at night be focused on the Lord, not on food.

I mentioned earlier that many people go to bed thinking about food, either looking forward to what they will eat tomorrow or lamenting with guilt and shame what they ate that day. Food is always on the minds of some people. I remember praying, "God, let me go through just one day without thinking about my issues with food!" I realized that I was seeking my soul satisfaction in the wrong place, because even my prayers were focused on food and not on doing God's will in the world.

Food Is *Not* Your Relationship with Family or Friends

In addition to thinking that food can define a relationship with God, some people use food as a substitute for a healthy relationship with their families and/or their friends.

I have to tell you about a precious woman I met in a First Place 4 Health class a few years ago. She came to realize that in spite of the wonderful family that God had given her, she was using fast-food restaurants as her family. When she had a problem she could not solve, she would run down to Uncle Mac and see what he had to offer; when she had something to celebrate, she would seek out big sister Wendy; and when she felt hormonal, she turned to dear old Aunt Arby! When she came to realize the role fast food was playing in her life, she finally began to experience real success. Now, after 30 years of fighting obesity, she has been successful and has reached her wellness goals.

Have you ever sought food when a significant relationship in your life began to fall apart? Have you ever sought solace with Ben and Jerry instead of a friend who could offer real support and a listening ear? The Body of Christ can be an excellent resource for you to draw from to develop good, honest relationships with others who will support you in your time of need. If you already have a church home with friends, talk with some of them about forming a support group. Then, on those days when you feel like diving into a big bag of potato chips because your emotions are ramped up, you can instead call a true friend for a good conversation and a nice walk.

Remember that "a friend loves at all times, and a brother is born for adversity" (Prov. 17:17). I can guarantee that the next time you are going through a difficult time, if you call a friend who has your best interest at heart instead of Uncle Mac, you'll feel the love that the Lord intends for you.

Food Is *Not* Your Comforter

Closely related to our using food as our families and/or friends is the misunderstanding that food can somehow create in us a sense of peace or happiness. While food can at times bring comfort, ultimately it does not bring the hope and support we need in difficult situations.

Do we really think that food can solve all of our problems? That "all you can eat" will be "all you will need"? I just heard a new tagline for an all-you-can-eat buffet: "Help yourself to happiness." I went to this buffet, and I will tell you what: The people eating there did not look happy! In fact, they looked miserable and almost resigned to getting third and fourth helpings.

So, where do we find our ultimate comfort? Jesus knew our need for comfort through difficult times; so, on the evening before He was crucified, He shared a wonderful meal with His disciples and then said these words: "I will ask the Father, and he will give you another Counselor to be with you forever—the Spirit of truth" (John 14:16-17). He sent a Comforter to be with us at all times.

The Holy Spirit stands with you and can speak to God on your behalf when you don't know what to say (see Rom. 8:26). Our comfort comes from knowing that the One who stands with us is God's gift to us to meet our deepest needs. Like an ultimate mentor, He is there to give us instructions about how to live.

You have been given an amazing gift in God's presence. If you ask Him to be with you in all things and you seek Him through prayer, you will find the comfort and peace you've been looking for in the freezer or at the fast-food window late at night. My greatest hope for you is that you'll come to know the Lord personally and that you'll experience His amazing power to help you live your best life for the rest of your life.

Tips for Avoiding Emotional Eating

If you've lived through a lifetime of eating to satisfy your emotions, it will take time to break that habit. Many of us began to overeat to meet a deeper need for acceptance and love when we were children, and breaking such a long-held pattern will be tough—but not impossible! Remember that all things are possible for those who believe and who begin to practice good habits.

To help you along your way to a new relationship with food, here are the top 10 ways to avoid unhealthy emotional eating:

1. If you can't get food out of your thoughts, drink something satisfying and wait 30 minutes. If the food craving passes, then you weren't really hungry.
2. If you typically snack at specific times of the day or after specific occasions, change your routine.
3. You will tend to eat less if you don't combine eating with another activity, such as watching television.
5. If too many hours pass between meals or snacks, your blood sugar will plummet and you will be more likely to overeat. So eat before you feel famished.
6. Pray through your favorite Scripture verses about food, self-control and your body as a "temple" every day.
7. Identify the locations where you are most likely to eat when you're feeling stressed, and avoid those places on busy or chaotic days. If you usually eat while driving, chew some gum instead or sip a bottle of water or a non-caloric beverage.
8. Keep a daily record of what you eat and review it before each meal. When you're aware of what you've already eaten that day, you may choose to forego that extra helping or sweet. Doing this before you eat will help you form the good habit of thinking before you eat.
9. If you have a pattern of snacking at a certain time of day, keep yourself occupied during that period.
10. Practice eating only when you're sitting down and when you're not otherwise occupied. This will allow you to savor your food and be mindful about what you are eating.

Remember that 70 percent of whether you reach your fitness goals depends on what you eat. Today is the day to change some habits and to begin to feel the joy and strength of eating to live, not living to eat!

The Importance of Exercise

One of my favorite all-time excuses for not exercising came from a lady I met at a fitness conference in Pennsylvania a few years ago. She stayed after my seminar to ask me a few questions. She was having a hard time getting past a plateau in her weight loss. She had lost a few pounds but needed to lose a lot more.

My first question was, "What are you doing for exercise?" She answered that she did not exercise at all and that even if she did, it would be a waste of time. "How is that?" I asked. She explained that exercise did not work for any of the women in her family and that it must be something that "runs in her family." She then turned and introduced me to her very overweight mother and said, "Right, Mom?" Now, really!

I have talked about the winning combination of healthy eating and daily exercise, so let me now go into more detail about the second half of that combination. Two questions I've heard over and over again over the past 20 years are, "Can I lose weight without exercise?" and "Can I be a healthy person without exercise?" While the answers to those questions may not be simple, there is one question that is easy to answer: yes, exercise *really is* that important.

Top 12 Benefits of Exercise

Over the years, I've found study after study that point out the benefits of exercise. But even more important than reading about exercise is that I've actually seen countless people discover how much joy exercise brings to their lives, in both the long run and the short run. Your ability to enjoy life and your family and friends, as well as your ability to do basic tasks, will increase exponentially as you begin to get fit. To get you thinking and excited about the benefits of exercise, I have listed below my Top 12 benefits of exercise. As you read, make a mental note about which benefit you would most love to experience in your life.

Benefit #1: Exercise Is Good for Your Heart

As stated in the *First Place 4 Health Member's Guide*, "Even 30 minutes of moderate-intensity activity . . . most days of the week can help prevent heart disease. The heart muscle is essential for pumping oxygen-rich blood to your major muscle groups and organs. Not only does regular activity strengthen your heart muscle, it also lowers blood pressure, increases the good (or HDL) cholesterol, lowers the bad (or LDL) cholesterol, and enhances blood flow. These benefits reduce your risk of stroke, heart disease and high blood pressure. Amazingly, studies have shown that you can get the same benefit from three 10-minute bouts of moderate activity as you can from one 30-minute session."[1]

What would it take for you to take three 10-minute walks every day? Imagine waking up 10 minutes earlier and taking a brisk walk around the block before breakfast. Perhaps you could go for a 10-minute excursion in the middle of the day as a mental break from your work. I will guarantee that a 10-minute walk will do more to wake you up from the afternoon droop than any amount of coffee or candy. What about taking your spouse and the kids for a daily evening power walk to talk about the best part (or worst part) of your day? You'll not only be building your heart but you'll be building the very "heart" of your relationship with your family.

Or maybe you can use your three 10-minute walks as time by yourself in order to spend more time with the Lord in prayer. In the morning, pray for your family and friends as they begin their day. At lunch, pray for co-workers or others who are involved in your work. At night, take 10 minutes to walk and review your day with the Lord, giving Him thanks for what you experienced and praying for areas of need.

Discover your own simple ways to build your heart muscle, including your heart for God and your love for your family and friends. It's *all* good!

Benefit #2: Exercise Plays a Role in Preventing Cancer

While cancer is not always the death sentence it was years ago, the reality of this disease will touch your life in some way (if it hasn't already). Did you realize that 25 to 30 percent of all major cancers may be related to weight issues and lack of activity?[2] Regular activity helps lower the risk of cancers of the colon, prostate, uterine lining and breast.[3] Diet and lifestyle (stop smoking and wear your sunscreen!) also play huge roles in preventing cancer. While the Lord will ultimately determine the length of your life, you have the ability to choose the health of your life. So why not exercise to help prevent the possibility of getting cancer?

Benefit #3: Exercise Reduces the Risk for Developing Type-2 Diabetes

More than 17 million Americans have type-2 diabetes, which affects the way the body uses blood sugar. However, one hour of brisk walking each day can reduce the risk of type-2 diabetes by 34 percent.[4] Imagine: Just a one-hour walk each day will improve your health dramatically for a lifetime!

I know what you are thinking: *Where am I going to find an hour each day to walk when I barely have time to take a shower?!* Over the years, I've become creative in the ways I find time to exercise. How about instead of driving to take care of errands at the grocery store or drugstore, you walk (briskly) to the store instead? This is the best type of multitasking! Over the years, I've made a concerted effort to walk to the store when I only need a few items. In addition to getting my body in shape, I've found these breaks in the middle of the day slow me down long enough to enjoy the weather, see other people and spend some one-on-one time with the Lord. Oh yeah, it also saves gas!

If you live within a 10- to 20-minute walk from the local drug or grocery store, put the car keys away and start decreasing your risk of diabetes as well as increasing your enjoyment of all the other benefits of a great walk in the neighborhood.

Benefit #4: Exercise Promotes Weight Loss

It's no secret that exercise burns calories. Fitness expert Bob Greene, known for his work with Oprah Winfrey, often refers to activity as "the gift that keeps on giving." Why? It raises your metabolism for a few hours after you've stopped exercising; thus, the rate at which you burn calories will remain higher than normal. Research has shown that to have the greatest effect on weight loss, you need to reduce your caloric intake and increase your exercise. Move more and eat less. The type of exercise or activity is not nearly as important as being consistent.[5]

Over the years, I've watched many peoples' desires to eat better increase simply because they were exercising. Once you've exercised in the morning and you realize your metabolism is still burning calories, you'll be less likely to eat that donut at the office. Why? Because once you've made your first good choice, it's easier to make your second good choice.

Benefit #5: Exercise Improves Muscle Strength and Joint Function

You need to have a certain level of muscle strength for everyday activities such as walking and climbing stairs. Through strength training, you can increase not only your muscle strength and muscle mass but also your bone strength.[6] As an added benefit, you'll boost your body's ability to burn calories. We will talk about building strength in a later chapter, but in order to get your creativity going, let me suggest a couple of ways you can begin today to strengthen your muscles without a major change to your lifestyle or taking away time from other activities.

When you are lifting the groceries from the car or carrying something into the house, pick up the bag a couple of times, as if you were lifting a weight. Do 5 to 10 repetitions before you place what you're carrying on the counter. If you do that with each bag, you'll be increasing your strength and burning calories.

Always take the stairs. The elevator may save a minute or two, but the stairs could add years to your life. As you climb, you'll also be strengthening your knees and joints. And if you are walking in an area that has some obstacles, always take the road less traveled. I live near the ocean, so when I walk on the beach, I climb over the jetties. I like the feeling of using all of my muscles. If you have children or grandchildren, they'll love to follow you on this "new adventure."

And, yes, you can join a gym and use equipment. God has given us so many ways to get fit, so why not take advantage of at least one or two of them?

Benefit #6: Exercise Prevents Osteoporosis

As you do some of the simple strength-training activities mentioned above and combine them with a healthy calcium intake, you'll be building strong bones. Exercise with impact, such as running, walking and lifting weights, helps combat and even reverse osteoporosis.[7] Did you know that women who walk four or more hours each week have 41 percent fewer hip fractures than those who walk less than an hour a week?[8] What you do in your 30s, 40s and 50s will help you prevent painful experiences in your 60s, 70s and 80s!

Benefit #7: Exercise Provides Emotional Benefits

Physical activity has an effect on your body's norepinephrine and serotonin levels. These neurotransmitters are involved in how you react to daily events. Exercise also causes your body to release feel-good chemicals called "endorphins." It can help you de-stress and improve your mood.[9] Just think: Taking a break to do 5 to 10 push-ups while leaning against the kitchen counter could decrease your stress while you are preparing a meal. Instead of feeling frustrated by the continual call of "how long until dinner," which might normally bother you, you could respond with a kinder, gentler attitude and change the entire atmosphere in your home.

Benefit #8: Exercise Battles the Effects of Aging

As we've mentioned, studies suggest that the greatest threat to health is not the aging process but inactivity. In addition to warding off numerous chronic diseases, regular exercise slows down the degeneration of the central nervous system that leads to slower reaction times and poor coordination. In a Harvard study, men who burned at least 2,000 calories a week by walking, jogging, climbing stairs or playing sports lived one to two years longer on average than did those who burned fewer than 500 calories a week by exercising.[10]

Benefit #9: Exercise Promotes Brain Health
Exercise increases the flow of blood to the brain, just as it improves circulation to the heart and the rest of the body. Activity also stimulates the growth of nerve cells in the part of the brain involved in memory.[11]

Benefit #10: Exercise Prevents Colds
In one study, researchers from the University of Carolina found that people who exercised regularly were 23 percent less likely to get colds than those who exercised less. Moreover, when those who exercised got colds, the symptoms disappeared more quickly than those who did little exercise. Health experts believe that exercise spikes the immune system for a few hours each day, helping ward off colds.[12] While there may be no cure for the common cold, exercise certainly has a big impact on it!

Benefit #11: Exercise Improves Sleeping Patterns
As we've already discussed, rest and sleep are critical for your overall health. Exercise improves your ability to sleep. This is because physical activity releases endorphins, which we discussed earlier. For this reason, if you are having problems getting to sleep or if your sleep is typically interrupted, try to exercise at least three hours before bedtime for the best results.[13]

Benefit #12: Exercise Enhances Your Sex Life
How could we leave this out? Experts confirm that the fitter we are, the better our sex life will be. According to the American Council on Exercise, "Being physically active can be a natural Viagra

boost." Being fit improves libido, blood circulation and sexual function. It also may make you feel better about yourself and, as a result, more sexually interested.[14]

Which Is Most Important?

Now, you tell me, which from the list above is the most important to you? You will have to decide if any of these benefits are valuable enough to you to make the sacrifices necessary for exercise to become a permanent part of your life.

All of these are important in my life. Both my mother and father had cardiovascular heart disease, so benefit #1 is paramount. In addition to having a bad heart, my mom developed lung cancer and also had diabetes. I am predisposed to the three major life-threatening diseases that affect women. I also am in the early stages of developing osteoarthritis in both of my knees.

I cannot say enough about the benefits of exercise as a mood enhancer. Exercise keeps me sane most days, especially on days when my calendar is full of activities. On my busiest days, there are two things I cannot do without: my quiet time and exercise—and usually I can make my exercise an extension of my quiet time.

Brain Fit or Brain Fried?

Is your brain fit or fried? There are days when my mind is definitely fried, and it desperately wants to be fit! I have a really bad habit of fixing my oatmeal for breakfast and then walking around the house eating it. I remember one morning, I sat the oatmeal down somewhere and could not remember where I had left it. Occasionally I misplace my car keys or lose my cell phone, but when I lose my food, something is seriously wrong! My brain had been on information overload for several months, and I was feeling totally worn out. No wonder I was losing track of my food!

One of the most important benefits of exercise is its impact on brain function. As a fitness professional, I encourage people to keep their bodies fit, but I have come to realize that we need to be as intentional about brain fitness. There are several simple "exercises" you can do for your brain, and they are not that hard—you can do them all and barely work up a sweat! Here are a few things that I do:

- *Maintain a connection with others.* People with an active social life can actually reduce the risk of dementia. We were not designed to live life by ourselves, but sometimes we get busy and act so self-sufficient that we wake up one morning to find that we have no one in our lives to stimulate our thinking! I need a lot of people in my life. I have friends with whom I pray, another group with whom I exercise, and another group with whom I connect on a daily basis. My friends help me see things in a different light and from a different perspective.

- *Keep learning.* Every time you learn something new, you develop new brain connections. I love my in-laws: They are retired Southern Baptist ministers, both over 80 years old, and amazing learners. I've been delighted when my husband, Rob, talks to his Dad, telling him about a new book he has just read and Papa says, "Oh yes, I finished that one myself last month." They never cease to amaze me! This year, consider signing up for a course or lessons in something that piques your interest. Try a community college or your local parks and recreation department.

- *Turn off the TV.* New studies show that people who watch more than seven hours of TV a day are at a higher risk of developing memory loss.[15] I would hate to add up all the hours in the lifetime of an average person that have been wasted by watching TV programs that had little or no eternal value.

- *Eliminate hurry from your life.* Nothing makes me crazier than having too much to do in my day. It causes my thinking to become frantic and unclear. I tend to make hasty and impulsive decisions when I am in a hurry. I make more mistakes and tend to forget things a lot more. When I have a lot to think about, I certainly don't need to have my decision-making process compromised. Having my prayer time every morning, and praying over my daily planner, helps me keep things in perspective. I ask God to prioritize my day so that it can unfold according to His plan for me.

• *Keep moving.* I can't begin to tell you how important exercise is in keeping the brain healthy: It helps with blood flow and improves mood. I have discovered that when my mind is bogged down with too much information, even a short walk will help clear it! In the end, I am not as concerned with the *length of my life* as much as I am with the *strength of my life.*

Common Questions About Exercising

Here are a few other common questions that I received from people about exercising.

Can I lose weight without exercise?

Yes, you can, but those who are most successful at keeping the weight off for more than five years almost always combine calorie control and exercise.

Can a person be healthy without exercise?

If you work at a job that requires a lot of physical labor, I would say yes; but the majority of Americans now primarily live a sedentary lifestyle.

What type of exercise should I do, and how long and hard should I exercise?

I recommend using the F.I.T.T. formula for exercise—Frequency, Intensity, Time and Type—as a guide to design a fitness program that fits your needs for each component of fitness (cardiovascular, strength-training and flexibility exercises). *Frequency* answers the question "How often should I exercise?" *Intensity* answers the question "How hard should I exercise?" *Time* answers the question "How long should I exercise?" *Type* answers the question "What kind of exercise should I do?" Answering each of these questions will lead to a balanced fitness program.

If exercise is so important, why didn't our ancestors exercise?

God designed our bodies for movement. We were not meant to be sedentary. Yet we have become a very sedentary society, to the point that we actually have to program in activities. Exercise is no longer just another part of our workday or home life as it was for our ancestors, so it no longer feels natural to our bodies. We are accustomed to sitting around.

There was a time in our society when there were no fitness clubs, because there was no need. I cannot imagine my grandmother having to program in activity to keep her healthy. She and my grandfather were farmers in east Tennessee and worked from sunup to sundown. Most of our ancestors worked at hard physical labor for a living. They would have never dreamed of going for a jog at the end of the day. They went to bed!

Not so for us. The majority of Americans do not work at physically challenging jobs, so we have to be very intentional about making sure we are physically active. Therefore, we need a plan. In the next three chapters, we are going to take a look at what a safe and balanced activity program looks like.

Things to Consider for a Balanced Fitness Plan

A balanced exercise program should include the following components:

1. Cardiovascular exercises
2. Muscular strength and endurance training exercises
3. Stretching and flexibility exercises
4. Healthy BMI

Cardiovascular exercises strengthen your lungs and heart and enhance weight loss by helping you burn calories. *Strength training* exercises promote muscular strength and endurance, help prevent injury, and increase lean-muscle mass. It can improve your strength and posture, reduce the risk of lower-back injury and help you stay toned. *Stretching and flexibility* exercises are needed to maintain joint range of motion and reduce the risk of injury and muscle soreness. Your *BMI* (body mass index) is a measure of body fat based on height and weight that applies to both adult men and women.[16]

Before we get started, let me say a word about having a healthy BMI. When you begin any wellness program, it will be helpful for you to know where you are. There are some basic standard measures for determining how healthy a person is, and one of those standards is your BMI.

BMI (body mass index) is the ratio of weight to height and is a rough but reliable indicator of body fatness (BMI does not measure body fat directly). BMI has become a key parameter in classifying overweight and obesity. You can calculate your own BMI by dividing your weight in pounds by your height in inches squared, and then multiply that result by a conversion factor of 703.[17] Here is an example for a person who is 5'10" and weighs 180 pounds:

- First, convert the height to inches. In this case, the person is 70 inches tall: (5 × 12) + 10.
- Multiply the result by itself to get the height squared: 70 × 70 = 4,900 inches.
- Divide the person's weight by height squared: 180 ÷ 4,900 = 0.0367.
- Multiply that number by 703: 0.0367 × 703 = 25.81.
- The person's BMI number is **25.81**.

Now calculate the BMI for your body:

- My height, converted to inches: _____
- That number multiplied by itself: _____
  (height squared)

- My weight: _____
- My weight divided by my height squared: _____
- That number x 703: _____
- My BMI: _____

Now use the following table to interpret your BMI:

BMI	Weight Status
Below 18.5	Underweight
18.5–24.9	Normal
25.0–29.9	Overweight
30.0–39.9	Obese
40.0 and above	Extreme Obesity

Because weight is not the only measure of health, I would encourage you to make an appointment with your doctor to get a comprehensive physical evaluation, including measures of your blood pressure and blood lipid levels, glucose tolerance testing, and other diagnostic tests your doctor may feel that you need.

Top 10 Tips for Nutritional Fitness

To achieve a healthy BMI, we need to stop overfeeding our bodies, so we need to look at the ways to achieve nutritional fitness. Below are simple things you can do that are proven tips for success in regard to nutrition and healthy eating. These are what we in First Place 4 Health call the Nutrition Top 10.[18]

1. *Set realistic and different goals.* Embrace the reality that your weight-loss journey will take much longer than just a few weeks—you want to plan to lose no more than two pounds a week—and set your goals accordingly. Also, set goals that focus on more than just the numbers on a scale. Are you physically stronger as the

result of your increased physical activity? Do you have more energy during the day? Have you seen other health benefits as a result of your efforts? Consider all of these factors when setting goals.

2. *Plan ahead and prioritize.* If you truly want to make your health a high priority, you must be intentional about preparing your environment to be a safe haven for healthy eating. Clear out junk food or any other barriers from your home, office or car that might hinder your efforts. To accomplish your goals, you must have a plan that makes sense to you and that you will relentlessly follow.

3. *Concentrate on quality.* Instead of labeling foods "good" or "bad," focus on what is the best food choice for you so you can reap the benefits. For instance, choose whole-grain bread over white bread. Look for foods with lots of fiber and choose fruits and vegetables over sweets. Select trim meats to cut out fat from your diet. Also choose low-fat milk (skim or 1%) and milk products, and be sure you choose enough calcium-rich foods.

4. *Quantity counts.* Eating too much of anything—whether it is healthy or unhealthy—can lead to weight gain. For this reason, you need to find a portion size that is appropriate for you. Practice reading labels and measuring out food portions until you feel you can make accurate educated guesses. Quit super-sizing, and try to cut your portions in half when eating at restaurants.

5. *Begin with a healthy breakfast.* When you get up in the morning, your glucose (blood sugar) level will be at its lowest of the day. For this reason, starting your day with a good breakfast within four hours after waking up will boost your energy levels and increase your attention span. In addition, studies show that people who eat breakfast generally burn

4 to 6 percent more calories than those who don't and eat fewer calories throughout the day!

6. *Choose better beverages.* Beverages supply nearly a quarter of Americans' total calories, and the largest contributors of these calories are nutrient-poor, sweetened beverages. For this reason, it is once again important to *choose* the healthier food option. In this case, choose water or calorie-free beverages in place of these sugary, high-calorie drinks. Low-fat milk and 100-percent fruit juice are also excellent substitutions.

7. *Spread your calories around.* Don't bunch all of your snacks and meals together. Instead, take your estimated calorie level and divide it by three meals and two snacks, and then eat these meals or snacks every three to five hours throughout the day (or every two to three hours or so if you're dealing with control of blood-sugar levels). When you plan in this manner, you will know when you will be eating again, and you won't have to wait until your stomach is growling. If possible, try to get the majority of your calories in by mid-afternoon and end the day with a lighter dinner.

8. *Balance your plate.* The U.S. Department of Agriculture (USDA) now uses a food plate in place of the food pyramid to illustrate the different foods groups you should be eating each day (see www.choosemyplate.gov). To balance your "food plate," divide every meal and snack into *quality* carbohydrates, proteins and fats in the appropriate *quantities* (see numbers 3 and 4 above). A few examples of balanced snacks would include fruit, nuts and yogurt; hummus, cheese and crackers; apple and peanut butter; and berries and cottage cheese.

9. *Read food labels.* Since 1965, all food products sold in the United States have required a label telling con-

sumers what is in the product and its nutritional properties. Nutrition facts are also provided at most restaurants and are even available online. Everything you need to know to make an informed decision about your food choices can be found by simply flipping the item over and reading this label.

10. *Practice mindfulness.* In a recent study conducted by Kaiser Permanente, participants who kept track of what they ate throughout the day had a success rate of meeting their goals nearly double of those who did not.[19] Writing down your food choices will make you more aware of your motivations and choices and will remind you to eat slowly and savor your meals.

Use these tips to develop your strategy for establishing a healthy relationship with food.

Getting Started with Exercise

In writing to the church in Philippi, the apostle Paul wrote this about the Christian life:

> Brothers, I do not consider myself yet to have taken hold of it [Christ's goal for me]. But one thing I do: Forgetting what is behind and straining toward what is ahead, I press on toward the goal to win the prize for which God has called me heavenward in Christ Jesus (Phil. 3:13-14).

What a powerful image of the Christian faith! Paul paints a picture of a runner who is straining forward to win, not worried about the past but simply looking toward the goal.

I invite you to have the same image in your plan for getting fit. The past is past. Now is the time to set that aside and choose a new way. It's time to set a long-term goal of incorporating physical activity into your lifestyle. Changing your lifestyle may seem overwhelming at first, but remember, you do not need to add the components of a fitness plan all at once. Too much, too fast, too soon will lead to the number three reason most people quit: burnout, which we want to avoid. In the next three chapters, we will examine how to develop a safe and effective exercise plan that you can stick to for the rest of your life.

Heart Care and Healthy Body Mass Index (BMI)

When someone who has not been exercising for a while decides it's finally time to get back in shape, one of the first questions that needs to be asked is, How's your heart? Sometime the reason we are out of shape is not the direct result of a physical problem. Sometimes a problem we're having manifests itself in our bodies, and we discover that our being overweight is really the result of a heart condition.

How's Your Heart?

The heart literally impacts every part of your exercise program. If your heart is strong and healthy, you'll be able to progress quickly toward your weight-loss goals. If you have a weak heart, then you'll need to move slowly at first until you build up this vital muscle.

When I begin to design an exercise program for someone, I consider his or her overall health. I ask, "How's your heart?" I want to know so much more than the person's resting heart rate or blood pressure. I want to know about his or her whole self.

One of the core principles at First Place 4 Health involves what we call the four-sided person. We've learned over the years that if we simply address someone's weight goals or exercise program, we've only helped one part of his or her overall health. In addition to the physical aspects of life, however, we also need to address the mental, spiritual and emotional aspects of each person. It's relatively easy to develop an exercise plan; the greater challenge is to understand the needs in a person's heart.

My friend Karen Creighton came to my First Place 4 Health class in the year 2000. She did not have a lot of weight to lose, but she was ready to make some changes in her life. Coming out of a marriage and raising two young daughters on her own, she did not feel very good about herself. What Karen discovered about herself was really a heart condition. Here is her story in her words:

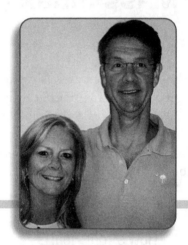

KAREN AND PAUL

Several years ago my life changed dramatically. I was deeply hurt by a relationship and desperately needed a new focus in my life. I was introduced by a friend to a Christ-centered health program called First Place 4 Health. This program came with several commitments, including exercise, spending time with God and other Christians, and eating healthy. I took the exercise commitment seriously and began with running.

Then I chose to join a Body & Soul Fitness class, which consisted of cardio and strength training. From there I went on to become a Body & Soul Fitness instructor and run marathons as well as compete in triathlons. I wanted my body to be strong for God. He worked in my life to help me overcome relational bondage that had control over my life. He changed my heart to become more like His. He also worked in my heart to help me strive to be a woman of excellence. I gave Him first place in my life, and everything else came next. Through First Place 4 Health and Body & Soul Fitness, God changed my heart as well as my body.

I am blessed now to be married to a man who has a heart for God and is someone who cares for me deeply. We have a blended family and have been married for eight years. Paul is my best friend, and we spend our free time exercising and traveling together. I am so thankful to have Paul in my life. Throughout the years, I have become much more disciplined in my spiritual walk as well as in my physical activities. The Lord continues to work in my life every day, helping me achieve balance with nutritional habits, exercise discipline and my devotion time spent with Him. I have been so thankful to be able to maintain this lifestyle over the years.

Throughout history, the heart has been considered the vital center and source of one's being, emotions and sensibilities. It is the root of our desires and values. When the Lord called His people to set priorities, He said, "Hear, O Israel, the LORD our God, the LORD is one. Love the LORD your God with all *your heart* and with all your soul and with all your strength" (Deut. 6:4-5, emphasis added).

A lifetime of wellness will require a wholehearted commitment. When we half-heartedly commit to something, it is doomed to fail. When our "hearts are not in it," we won't have the enthusiasm necessary to be successful, and we may not follow through.

The heart contains our deepest and sincerest feelings and beliefs and is the seat of our intellect and imagination. In fact, one of the core principles of wisdom in Scripture is to allow God's Word to dwell in our hearts, because it's out of a healthy heart that we'll find a life that is like a well full of water. As Proverbs 4:20-23 states:

> My son, pay attention to what I say; listen closely to my words. Do not let them out of your sight, keep them within your heart; for they are life to those who find them and health to a man's whole body. Above all else, guard your heart, for it is the wellspring of life.

The state of God's heart permeates the entire story of the Bible. From Genesis to Revelation, the Lord inquires about the state of the heart of those who seek to follow or not follow Him. Scripture refers to the heart more than 740 times.

Who Holds Your Heart?

After years of struggle in the desert, after years of wandering and years of fighting battles, God's Chosen People were ready to settle into the land He had promised to their ancestor Abraham. A relative peace had been established, and Joshua called all the tribes together to encourage and challenge the people to keep their hearts set on God. As he challenged the crowds to follow the Lord, they shouted with one voice that they intended to follow the Lord only:

> Then Joshua said, "You are witnesses against yourselves that you have chosen to serve the LORD."
> "Yes, we are witnesses," they replied.
> "Now then," said Joshua, "throw away the foreign gods that are among you and *yield your hearts to the LORD*, the God of Israel."
> And the people said to Joshua, "We will serve the LORD our God and obey him" (Josh. 24:22-24, emphasis added).

Joshua knew that without a commitment—without a vow to place God first above all else—the people would likely turn away from God. In the same way, if we allow other gods to take hold of us, eventually our hearts will lose both strength and life. Like Solomon, Joshua knew that the people needed to guard their hearts.

So who holds your heart? When you look at your life, do you have a heart that is yielded to God and desires to follow His plan? Does your heart long for God's best in your life? If you are ready to get fit, then you'll need a heart that is yielded only to God.

How Do You Guard Your Heart?

Just as there are certain exercises you can do to strengthen your physical heart, there are spiritual exercises you can do to guard your spiritual heart. You'll be amazed at how a few simple, small steps can have a huge impact on your emotional, spiritual and physical wellbeing.

One of the greatest missionaries of the first century knew the importance of guarding the heart. Paul spent a lot of time in jail, getting beaten up and running from town to town (not for exercise!) in order to tell others about Jesus. How did he keep from getting discouraged? He lets us in on his secret in a letter he wrote to his friends in a city called Philippi:

> Do not be anxious about anything, but in everything, by prayer and petition, with thanksgiving, present your requests to God. And the peace of God, which transcends all understanding, will guard your hearts and your minds in Christ Jesus (Phil. 4:6-7).

Constant prayer and thanksgiving help guard our hearts. When we pray, we yield our hearts to God. When we give thanks for all our circumstances, we yield our minds to God. The anxiety, or stress, that causes our physical hearts to go bad is replaced with peace when our hearts and minds rest fully and completely in God's care.

During the time my oldest son was going through some rough days trying to find his way in life, I was tempted to let worry and anxiety rule my heart instead of God's truth. I was close to suffering an emotional heart attack. I continued to seek God through prayer and by meditating on His Word. I continued to give thanks for the day that Michael gave his heart to Jesus. Through these simple exercises, God continually calmed and strengthened my heart with His presence and His peace, and He delivered me from my emotional heart attack.

Finally, after giving God a year of his life, Michael came to the place where he is now: all in, with both feet, for Christ and His kingdom. Little did I know that the biggest challenge of my life would end up with God calling Michael to the mission field! Oh my heart! The mission field of his calling is in a faraway, rugged country. He is leaving to go there with his bride and my only grandchild (as of this writing). But my heart is not broken—my heart is hopeful and strong! God has protected my heart and fortified my heart with the love I have for my son.

As you can see, our hearts keep us going in so many more ways than simply pumping oxygen-rich blood to our vital organs. It holds so much more. Once we begin to address our "heart condition" spiritually, we are ready to address our physical heart through exercise, eating and rest.

Where Should You Start?

Anatomically speaking, the heart is "the hollow muscular organ in vertebrates whose contractions propel the blood through the circulatory system. In mammals it consists of a right and left atrium and a right and left ventricle."[1] We don't really think of the heart as a muscle, mostly because we can't see it. Most of the muscles on our skeleton are quite visible under the skin. As we work on these muscles, we can see visual results, usually within a few weeks. Not so with the heart. We really cannot see our hearts, but we *can* certainly feel them.

The Objective

Keeping the heart muscle strong and healthy is the main objective of cardiovascular exercise. A healthy heart will be able to pump oxygen-rich blood with one strong contraction. If upon exertion your heart beats really fast, it is making more contractions to get the blood to the vital organs. When you are jogging, for example, your legs are really going to need blood pumping into them, so a healthy heartbeat will be strong and get the blood flowing without much strain or without having to beat so many times to get the job done. Spiritually, it is vital that we keep our hearts pure and strong as we do physically. A pure heart is a healthy heart. A strong heart is a healthy heart.

The best and most effective way to strengthen your heart and lungs is with cardiovascular, or aerobic, activities. These are exercises that are strenuous enough to temporarily speed up your breathing and heart rate. While performing these activities, you will probably feel out of breath but not gasping for air. You should be able to carry on a conversation but not sing. Many people are fearful of getting their heart rate up, especially if they have not been exercising in a while or are out of condition. Some who are just beginners at exercise may be surprised by how their bodies feel after working in such a strong way.

I remember a precious Southern lady in one of my cardio classes. This was the first time she had ever exercised in her life. She was brought up in a well-to-do Kentucky family, and it was not ladylike to run or jump. She went to finishing school and was well schooled in all of the Southern social graces. She came that first day to my class with a darling outfit on (not exercise clothes, mind you) and her little white tennis shoes. After about 10 minutes she looked at me with panic in her eyes and hurried outside. I followed her and asked, "Miss Kathryn, what is wrong?" "I think I am having a heart attack!" I quickly checked her pulse and found it was beating quite fast but strong. "Are you having any pain?" "No," she said, "but my heart is just running away!" She had never gotten her heart rate up in 65 years!

Physical Evaluation

The first step in any workout routine is to evaluate how fit you are for your chosen physical activity. As I mentioned earlier, when you begin an exercise program, it's wise to consult a doctor. According to Dr. Cedric Bryant, chief exercise physiologist for the American Council on Exercise, this is especially true for anyone with major health risks, males aged 45 and older, and women aged 55 and older.[2]

In the almost 20 years that I have been teaching fitness, I cannot remember a time when someone who wanted to start an exercise program was not given the green light from their doctor to begin sensibly. Even with pre-existing medical conditions, you can usually work out in some way. Dr. Stephanie Siegrist, an orthopedic surgeon in private practice in Rochester, New York, says, "I can't think of any medical issue that would get worse from the right kind of exercise."[3]

Cardio Benefits

Cardiovascular activities (usually just called cardio) are designed to strengthen your heart and lungs. Your heart grows stronger as the exercise requires your heart to pump harder and faster to get the blood flowing and improve oxygen consumption. At the same time, your lungs are working harder too. An additional benefit of cardio is the excess calories that are burned off in the process—a vital part of weight management. The less weight you carry around, the less of an overload you place on your heart and lungs. Cardio exercises are also essential in lowering bad cholesterol and preventing many other diseases. As the variety, intensity and duration of activity increase, you will also experience many additional health benefits.

Cardio Activities

Cardiovascular endurance is the ability of your body's circulatory and respiratory systems to supply fuel during sustained physical activity. To strengthen your heart and lungs, try activities that keep your heart rate elevated at a safe level for a sustained length of time, such as walking, swimming or bicycling. To really get the maximum benefit from cardio exercises, choose exercises that involve your major muscle groups, such as your legs, arms and back. The activity you choose does not have to be strenuous to improve your cardiovascular endurance. Start slowly with an activity you enjoy and gradually increase the time and intensity.[4]

A walking to running program is probably one of the most time efficient and effective workouts. Walking and running have endured the test of time, require very little training or little equipment, and can be done just about anywhere. I know from personal experience that starting slowly is the best way to go because this is exactly how I got started more than 25 years ago. In high school I was a cheerleader, but I always wanted to be a runner. I did not think I had the endurance for it, but I started slowly and basically followed the step-by-step guidelines given on the following page. This is a chart recommended by the American Council on Exercise on how to get moving safely and without injury.

Once again, it is important to consult with your doctor before beginning any exercise program to determine whether running is appropriate for you. If you have orthopedic problems, heart problems, or are currently considered obese, you should probably bypass running in favor of walking.[6] Be patient with yourself and do not rush the progress. Nothing will derail your efforts at cardio exercises like traumatized hamstrings or knees!

Guidelines for Starting a Running Program[5]

Week	Time*	Intensity**
1	20 min.	Moderate-pace walk
2	22 min.	Moderate-to-brisk pace walk
3	22 min.	30-45 sec. jog, 5 min. walk (repeat 3x)
4	24 min.	45-60 sec. jog, 5 min. walk (repeat 3x)
5	24 min.	30-45 sec. jog, 4 min. walk (repeat 4x)
6	26 min.	45-60 sec. jog, 4 min. walk (repeat 4x)
7	26 min.	30-45 sec. jog, 3 min. walk (repeat 5x)
8	28 min.	45-60 sec. jog, 3 min. walk (repeat 5x)
9	28 min.	30-45 sec. jog, 2 min. walk (repeat 6x)
10	30 min.	45-60 sec. jog, 2 min. walk (repeat 6x)
11	30 min.	2 min. jog, 1 min. walk (repeat 6x)
12+	30 min.	Gradually progress to continuous jogging

* Total time includes 3-minute warm-up and 3-minute cool-down.

** Individuals who are in good shape may progress at a faster rate by increasing time and intensity simultaneously, while those who are less fit may opt to progress more gradually.

The F.I.T.T. formula for cardio exercises given below lists the details you need to know about starting a cardio fitness program.

- *Frequency:* 3 to 5 times each week. Increase this amount to five times or more each week to maximize weight loss.
- *Intensity:* 50 to 85 percent of target heart rate.
- *Time:* 20 to 60 minutes of continuous aerobic activity (minimum of 10-minute bouts accumulated throughout the day)
- *Type:* Activities that use large muscle groups that can be maintained continuously and are aerobic in nature, such as walking, jogging, swimming, biking and dancing.[7]

Motivation

In order to persist and be consistent with your cardio exercises, you will need to—you guessed it—identify a sustaining motivation. Look at each of the benefits to cardio exercises listed below, and then choose which one would best motivate you to stay focused on your goals:

- *Strengthen heart and lungs*—to be able to hike and climb with your children, grandchildren or friends.
- *Lower LDL cholesterol*—to get off cholesterol medications or never have to go on them in the first place!
- *Burn calories to lower body fat*—to fit comfortably in an airplane seat for a missions trip or to fit back into some of your favorite clothes.
- *Increase bone density*—to be strong enough to carry in the groceries, one bag in each hand, or be able to easily carry a grandchild.
- *Sense of wellbeing*—to be able to do what needs to be done and do it well!

So, How's Your Heart?

Remember my friend Karen, whose story I told near the beginning of the chapter? The cool thing about Karen is that she did not just lose the weight she needed but went way beyond that! God led her to become a fitness instructor with Body & Soul ministries, and she teaches fitness classes in the Charleston, South Carolina, area. Karen is also now a champion athlete, participating in triathlons and marathons. God did way more than Karen could have hoped for or imagined—during her training time Karen met her husband, Paul, who is also a stellar athlete. It's amazing what can happen when a person is totally yielded to the lordship of Christ spiritually, mentally and physically!

11

Strength Training

A couple of years ago, my friend Carole Lewis, National Director for First Place 4 Health, took a nasty fall from her bike. Just a week after that, she had an encounter with a dog leash that was attached to a very big dog. Knocked off her feet twice in a row, she was okay (amazingly!) and suffered nothing more than a couple of scrapes and bruises. A less-fit woman would have broken a hip or shoulder. In fact, according to recent studies, one out of three adults 65 years and older experiences a fall each year, and in most cases, the fall will result in a head injury, a hip fracture or even, in some cases, an early death.[1] Other statistics are just as alarming:

- In 2007, more than 18,000 older adults died from unintentional fall injuries.[2]
- The death rates from falls among older men and women have risen sharply during the past decade.[3]
- In 2009, 2.2 million nonfatal fall injuries among older adults were treated in emergency departments, and more than 581,000 of these patients were hospitalized.[4]

What made the difference for Carole? Two powerful words: "strength training." The sad truth is that most of the falls that made up these statistics either could have been prevented, or the extent of the injuries could have been dramatically less if strength training had been a regular part of daily activity. While there is no question that Carole is an amazing woman, her lifestyle of regularly taking care of her body and building her muscles prepared her to survive and thrive despite the accidents.

Do you want to be healthy as long as you live? A regular discipline of strength training will help you to not only live longer but also live better.

Strength Training in the Bible

One of my favorite strongmen of the Bible is Caleb. You may remember Caleb from the book of Numbers. As part of the group of people who were led by Moses out of slavery in Egypt and into the Promised Land, Caleb had a spirit that was different from most. When the people arrived at the land the Lord had promised them, Moses sent 12 spies to check out the land and see what kind of people already lived there. When the 12 men returned, 10 were completely discouraged, beaten down and convinced that Moses (and the Lord) had made a mistake. They reported that the people living in the land were GIANTS! They were warriors and were not going to simply hand their land over to these new arrivals.

While the 10 other spies were trying to convince the people to give up before they even started, Caleb and Joshua believed that the Lord would give them the land. Caleb and Joshua had confidence in God's ability to follow through on His promises, and they were ready to fight. They told the people, "Do not be afraid of the people of the land, because we will swallow them up. Their protection is gone, but the LORD is with us. Do not be afraid of them" (Num. 14:9).

Caleb saw a challenge, he saw the Lord's favor, and he was ready to overcome. His courage and faith inspire me: When I face new and difficult opportunities, I think of Caleb's absolute confidence in God's provision. Unfortunately, he and Joshua were not able to inspire the people of Israel—the people continued to complain until eventually the Lord led them back into the desert. In fact, with the exception of Caleb and Joshua, none of the adults who were originally promised the land lived to set foot on it (they died in the desert), so the Lord gave the land to their children 40 years later. I wonder how many times we have missed out on God's promises because we refused to trust His ability to lead and carry us through difficult tasks. If we are willing to sacrifice and trust God, anything is possible.

When Joshua and the people returned to Canaan a second time, they were ready to take the land. Forty years in the desert can have that kind of impact on a person! Evidently, the Chosen People had finally grown tired of living lives that were less fulfilling than what God wanted to give them. After years of fighting, they conquered most of the territory that God had promised, with the exception of the hill country in which the giants (called the sons of Anak) dwelled. These were the giants who had caused such great fear 40 years earlier. The people of Israel were still not able to penetrate their stronghold.

Guess who took up the challenge? Of course, it was Caleb. Listen to these inspiring words from a man well into his 80s:

> Now then, just as the LORD promised, he has kept me alive for forty-five years since the time he said this to Moses, while Israel moved about in the desert. So here I am today, eighty-five years old! I am still as strong today as the day Moses sent me out; I'm just as vigorous to go out to battle now as I was then. Now give me this hill country that the LORD promised me that day. You yourself heard then that the Anakites were there and their cities were large and fortified, but, the LORD helping me, I will drive them out just as he said (Josh. 14:10-12).

Wow! Caleb had spent his lifetime staying strong both in body and in faith. At 85, he was ready to take on challenges that men half his age would not even consider. A life of strength training and trusting God had prepared him for his greatest challenge. Likewise, if you want to be able to face your giants—even when you are well into your 80s—strength training (both in body and prayer) will prepare you to receive God's best for you.

Joshua is another strongman in the Bible. He had inherited an impossible job. The Lord had called him to lead a group of people who were untrained for war and had spent most of their lives in the desert to invade a land of people who were like giants and well situated behind walls in fortified cities. In fact, the first city Joshua and the Chosen People faced was Jericho, which had never been conquered because of the huge walls around the city. Joshua needed encouragement, and the Lord spoke powerful words into his life. As you begin to take up the challenge of what might seem like an impossible task toward a life of wellness, allow these words to bring you encouragement and inspiration to face your next greatest challenge:

> The Lord said to Joshua, "Be strong and courageous, because you will lead these people to inherit the land I swore to their forefathers to give them. Be strong and very courageous. Be careful to obey all the law my servant Moses gave you; do not turn from the right or to the left, that you may be successful wherever you go" (Josh. 1:6-7).

How did Joshua respond? He immediately began to make plans to follow God's best. With the confidence of Caleb, Joshua told the people to start getting ready, because in three days, they would confront the walls that stood in the way of experiencing God's best for their lives.

Benefits of Strength Training

Strength training can definitely improve our quality of life as we grow older, but it's good for us at any age. When my mom passed away, we had a big estate sale to get rid of all of the things that none of us wanted and were even difficult to give away. The entire family gathered at the old home and started carrying out the bounty into the front yard. There were probably 10 of us there: me and my sister; my 23-year-old son, Mark; and lots of male cousins. The funny thing was that when it came to the heavy lifting, Mark and I were the only ones able to do it!

One male cousin supervised because of his "bad back," and there were two others on strict doctors' orders not to do any heavy lifting (one due to a recent heart attack and the other due to a blood-pressure problem). So that left me and Mark! We carried out wall units and most everything that was heavy. At the time it was really funny: There I was, "just a girl," helping to do all the heavy lifting! The other guys should have been embarrassed. How grateful I was (and am!) that I am strong and that I have continued to work hard to maintain my strength over the years by lifting weights. You may not think you are muscular, but you are. Your body contains more than 600 muscles, and together they account for one-third to one-half of your body weight. As children and young men and women we have all the muscle we need, but starting at around age 40, most of us lose nearly half a pound of muscle each year. At the same time, we gain the same amount of fat, so that by age 80 we have only about one-third of the muscle we had when we were 40. But here's the great news: You don't have to lose muscle and gain fat! You, like Carole or Caleb, can live a life of strength training that will have tremendous benefits today and in the future.

Reasons to Strength Train

As I've continued to study, work with others and experience weight training in my own life, I've discovered eight compelling reasons to pursue strength training on a regular basis. As you consider these reasons, think about which one would motivate you to start a program of strength training for yourself.

1. *Strength training helps combat osteoporosis.* When you "stress" your skeletal muscles, you "stress" your skeleton. Bones become stronger and denser, as do the surrounding muscles.

2. *Strength training helps combat age-related problems and degenerative diseases that contribute to the "aging" of our bodies.* Much of the bone and muscle loss that we attribute to aging is actually caused by lack of use.

3. *Strength training helps you tone.* Lean muscle weighs more than fat, but it takes up less space. As you develop strength, take your body measurements and be encouraged! Remember that muscle is the primary calorie burner. Because muscle tissue is active tissue and consumes

calories, the more lean body tissue you have, the more calories you burn all day long!

4. *Strength training helps rehabilitate muscle.* Strength training helps to build previously injured or weak muscle groups by increasing range of motion and strengthening connective tissue.

5. *Strength training can help correct muscle imbalances.* Two-thirds of all our muscles are located above our waist and are hardly touched by many popular aerobic activities.

6. *Strength training provides extra abdominal work.* When the abdominals are properly used to stabilize the torso during many weight-bearing exercises, your abdominal muscles get an extra workout.

7. *Strength training makes many activities in everyday life easier.* This is "practical fitness" as you go about your activities of daily living, such as lifting heavy grocery bags, picking up babies, moving furniture, and so forth. The stronger you are, the easier it is to move, and the more you will accomplish.[5]

8. *Strength training lifts depression by lifting our spirits and increasing our overall confidence with being and feeling stronger.*[6] Imagine Caleb at 85 giving an inspirational talk at your church or company about taking on the giants. As you develop your strength training, you'll be amazed by how much better you'll feel about work, your relationships, dealing with others (young and old), and playing sports or running errands.

Muscles are not only beautiful to look at but are fascinating in function as well. Muscle is composed of two fiber types: fast twitch and slow twitch. Fast-twitch fibers contract very quickly and explosively; they give the body power. Slow-twitch fibers contract more slowly and with more control; they give the body endurance.

Cardiovascular workouts help us develop slow-twitch muscle fibers. By adding strength training, we will help develop our fast-twitch fibers, especially as we challenge our bodies appropriately with heavier weights.

The How and How Much of Strength Training

The American College of Sports Medicine (ACSM) recommends a minimum of two sessions of strength training per week. These strength-training sessions are in addition to the three or four sessions of cardio exercise per week that the ACSM recommends.[7] How much you get out of your strength-training workout is determined by three factors:

1. The number of times each movement is repeated (number of reps)
2. The speed of each movement
3. The size of the weights or amount of resistance used

To train for strength rather than endurance, use *slower movements* and *heavier weights* or *stronger resistance bands*. (Note: Because women have different hormone levels than men, it is unlikely that women will see a dramatic increase in muscle size.) Select weights that are heavy enough to be a challenge. Strict strength training actually takes the muscle "to failure." This means that you cannot do another rep using proper form. Weights should be heavy enough that it is difficult to get through the entire set. As training begins, it may be necessary to stop and rest rather than continue. This is especially true if you start to compromise your position and compensate with other muscle groups such as the neck and back.[8]

Tools of the Training
Here's what you need to get started:

- *Hand-held weights:* I recommend that you use hand-held weights for resistance. Work up to using five-pound

weights or more as quickly as possible to really experience the benefits of strength training. Even if you cannot do all the repetitions at first, you will see quick
improvement by challenging your muscles with heavier
weights. Keep in mind that strength is lost quickly if you
stop doing strength training (in other words, your muscles will atrophy). So after a sickness, holiday or time
away from strength training, you will need to build back
up to your former strength level. Consistency is extremely important in building lean muscle tissue.[9]

- *Resistance bands:* Resistance bands (such as Dyna-Bands®)
  are made of elastic and provide another effective method
  for strength training. Most fitness stores stock them in
  several resistance sizes. Bands provide dynamic resistance through the whole range of motion of each exercise
  and can be very effective for strength cross-training because they challenge the muscle groups in a different way
  than hand weights. When using bands, always make sure
  you control the band and move through each exercise
  movement slowly and in a controlled manner as the
  band provides external resistance.[10]

- *Your own body:* Using your own body as your resistance is
  one of the best ways to build strength. Push-ups, pull-
  ups, squats and lunges are all examples of body-resistance
  exercises and can be performed just about anywhere.

Easy Ways to Get Started

Here are a couple of simple ways to start the process of strength
training that will allow you to experience some of the benefits of
strength training without adding too much (initially) to your
workout.

When you are sitting down, never use your hand or arms to
help you get up, but simply use your legs. At first this might be a
challenge, but with practice, you'll be able to use your weight to

your advantage. Your present weight will actually become a "partner" in strengthening your leg muscles!

Push-ups, as I mentioned in an earlier chapter, can be done anywhere, using any surface to gauge your resistance. When talking to your spouse, why not use the kitchen chair to do 5 to 10 repetitions of push-ups? If you have children, you could even have a push-up challenge at the dining-room table before a meal. I've been known to do push-ups leaning against the kitchen sink while I put away dishes from the dishwasher.

Be creative. If you start with even small steps as you begin strength training, you'll be encouraged to take larger steps.

Guidelines to Follow

As you begin, you'll need to follow a couple of guidelines to make your time most effective. While there are not a lot of rules to follow when it comes to strength training, proper body alignment and posture will help prevent injury. Here are just a few tips:

- *Keep a tight core body (tighten the abdominals and gluteus muscles) with every rep.* Torso stabilization and good posture are the keys to proper alignment and execution of most strength-training movements.

- *Stop when you have performed all the reps you can do using proper form.* Proper body alignment is critical. Bad posture indicates fatigue. Do not compromise your position.

- *Avoid hyperextension and locking joints.* Be especially mindful of your elbows and knees. If you lock a joint, it means that the joint is holding the weight instead of the muscles. You are not building strength but are leaving yourself open to injury by stressing the joint.

- *Think "slow and controlled" through all movements.* Do not rush through any of the movements. Do not "heave" the weight so that you have to "brake" it at the end of the range of motion. Control the weight through the full range of motion.

- *Remember to breathe.* Exhale on exertion (when you are moving against gravity), and inhale on the release. Do not hold your breath, as this can raise blood pressure.

- *Work out at least two times per week.* The length of time for each session will vary and will depend on the number of muscle groups worked. Usually, a 30-minute session will be adequate time to target each muscle group. Doing strength training exercises only once each week is not often enough to achieve results. Three times a week may be even more effective; however, allow one day of rest between sessions so your muscles can recover.[11]

Have fun as you begin this part of your fitness plan. A word of warning, however: Many people get discouraged and lose their motivation within the first three weeks of strength training, so in order to help prevent that, keep your eyes on the Lord.

Taking a Hit

Just as we need strength and endurance physically, we need the same strength and endurance emotionally and spiritually as well. Many of us are continually getting knocked down by life, so we need to develop the inner strength that will keep us from giving up on ourselves and others. We need to learn how to take a hit.

Let's talk about hitting for a bit. I have three boys and one girl, so you can imagine there was a lot of hitting in my household when they were younger. I tried to teach them this principal:

We don't need to learn to hit; we need to learn how to take one.

All three of my sons played football. One played on the college level, and the other two had successful high school experiences. I clearly remember my oldest son wanting to play football when he got to high school. He had played soccer and basketball since he was a small boy, but I had never really encouraged him to play football. After all, it's so violent! I finally gave in, and he made the team.

Being a fitness person, I thought I would drop by the afternoon football practice to see if his coaches needed any help. Taking a seat in the bleachers, I decided it might be a good idea just to watch for a while before I started to tell the coaches my expert advice. What they were doing that day was called hitting practice, which sounds horrible—as a mom, I had tried to have what I called no-hitting practice. Anyway, on the practice field, the coach would blow the whistle and they would all go after one guy!

Later that day, I asked Michael, the coach, "What was the point of getting knocked down to the ground, time after time? Were you trying to teach the players how to not get knocked down?" "No, not at all," he said. "In football there is no way to avoid getting knocked down. The point of the drill was to teach the team how to get back up. It's a valuable lesson because it helps you get strong and learn not to be afraid of the hits that are bound to come." After watching hundreds of football games, I now realize that our real strength is demonstrated when we get back up after we've been hit; that shows inner and outer strength.

The ability to take a hit has an amazing impact on the world around us. We have all seen it. We're watching a game and, suddenly, one of the players takes a hard hit—so hard that you can even hear it. It causes the crowd to wince in sympathy. (As a mom I hate that sound!) And we wait, wait . . . for what? For the player to get up! And when the player gets up, what is our response? We cheer!

Getting up after taking a hit is exactly what the coach and the fans want to see. And it's what God wants us to do in our everyday lives too.

One of the most impressive testimonies I've ever heard about taking a hit comes from Dawn Bland. When Dawn joined First Place 4 Health she was motivated, but as you'll learn, God was preparing her for a tremendous hit.

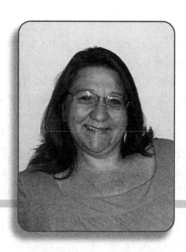

DAWN BLAND

Friedrich Nietzsche wrote, "What does not kill me makes me stronger." These words have inspired me over the years as I've improved my physical strength, beginning in 1996.

I have always loved to dance and praise God, so joining the Body & Soul Fitness class at Remount Baptist Church was perfect for me. Even as a heavier person, I have always known how important exercise is to my body. I've always wanted to be strong and healthy. The dancing part of the class was really fun, but the strength training was hard work. Little did I know just how beneficial this strength would become.

On Sunday, September 29, 2002, I was involved in a car accident. My son was driving and we were struck on the passenger side, by a car going 60 miles an hour. I was the passenger. Paramedics worked fast to get me out of the car and get me to the nearest hospital. After I was stabilized, I was flown by helicopter to a trauma unit. My pelvis was broken in three places, and my tailbone was broken in two places. My liver was lacerated, and I was bleeding internally. All the ribs on my right side were broken, my lungs had collapsed, and my right shoulder was completely separated at the socket. My eyes had also been burned by radiator fluid and battery acid. Things did not look good for me.

The main thing the doctor was concerned about was my liver. It was severely lacerated, and they were giving me blood platelets to help clot the blood. The last thing he wanted to do was to take me into surgery at that time, because I most likely would not pull through. He was even afraid I might not make it through the night. For the next three days, all anyone could do was pray.

They could not get the bleeding to stop, and my lungs collapsed a total of three times. I was on a respirator, and I was given transfusions because of the bleeding in my liver. Tubes had been placed in my lungs to drain the fluid. On Friday, October 4, not quite a week after the accident, I was strong enough to leave the ICU and go into surgery. A metal rod was placed in my hip to put the bone back together, and after surgery I was placed in the step-down unit to recover.

By Wednesday, October 9, my doctors were saying, "You are a miracle. We have never seen anyone recover as fast or as well as you are." I said, "That's the power of prayer and because God is a good God!" They said if I continued to do well, I would be able to leave the hospital on Friday, October 11. One week after my surgery I was able to go home.

Recovery was not easy. Every day I would tell myself, One day this pain will go away. One day I will wake up and the pain won't be so bad. I can do this! Each time I would go to the doctor, he would be amazed at how well I was doing. By the first of December, the doctor said, "Well, I can't believe this, but I think you are ready to start putting pressure on your right leg and start learning to walk on it." Because my injuries were so severe, the doctor had not expected me to be able to use my leg for almost three months. He said, "Mrs. Bland, you are a medical miracle. We can't explain it, but you're doing better than we ever expected." I told him that was the power of God, healthy eating, and exercise. He certainly agreed.

By December of that year, I was walking with a walker. By January 2003, I was walking with a cane and then on my own with no help at all. When I started my physical therapy, they kept telling me to slow down and take it easy. They could not believe how quickly I was recovering. I told them I had been exercising and taking part in an exercise and spiritual program called Body & Soul for years.

Now I tell people that I would not be here if it were not for the grace of God and being so strong and healthy. I overcame my injuries because of God's grace and because I had a strong body. All those years of Body & Soul Fitness classes, combined with all those years of walking with my Lord, gave me the strength I needed to pull through one of the toughest times of my life.

I stand today strong, whole and living life to its fullest.

Are You Ready to Get Strong?

Can you take a hit? Sometimes I feel as if I get knocked down every day. I try so hard to avoid the hits, but they just keep coming. Some days I feel as though I am recklessly dodging bullets from every direction. I get mad, I pout, I stomp my feet, and I struggle. I try with all my might to be a good mom, to be a good wife, to be a good pastor's wife for my church, to protect my kids—but I sometimes get hit so hard that the ball flies past me or, worse than that, I totally drop the ball.

Satan has such victory over me sometimes, and he knows just where to hit me to make me hurt the most. As a result, his hits usually drive me to my knees and leave me feeling humiliated, defeated and helpless. It happened to me just today when I thought I would be unable to finish this book—that I did not have the strength, knowledge or wherewithal to complete the task.

Then my Father—the Lion of Judah, the Ancient of Days, the Star of David, the Giver of every good and perfect gift—rushed into my life and lifted me up out of the miry clay and placed my feet on a solid rock. He put a new song in my heart and whispered in my ear, "My grace is sufficient. I will make myself strong in you. I will finish the good work I started with this book." He did what He said He would do, right in the face of my enemy and in front of this old, mean world.

It's through the hits I have taken in life that I have learned the great reality of God's love and strength. The important point to remember is that winning at wellness must be intentional—it does not happen by accident. If you truly desire the strength of the Lord Jesus Christ, He will give it to you. And if you have that, you cannot fail. So get up and let's keep going!

12

Flexibility and Stretching

Climbing walls—I've always been fascinated and a little intimidated by them. You could say that I've been intrigued from a distance, and I figured one day I would get my chance to climb a wall and make it to the top. Well, while I was attending Wellness Week at Sandy Cove retreat center, I had my opportunity.

With excitement and a little fear, I took on the challenge of climbing the wall. If you've never climbed a wall, let me tell you right now, it is way harder than it looks! I started out pretty strong and made my way up about 15 feet, when I started to get really tired. I felt as though I had used every muscle group just to make the first 15 feet. I had about 20 more feet to go before the top. Pushing on, I came to a spot where I just could not find a handhold. Every hold I tried was just a little out of reach for me. I told the Lord, "If You only had given me another inch, I could reach this next one and, besides that, I would be at my perfect weight!"

I tried moving a little to the left and then to the right. No luck. No matter where I positioned myself, I could not get to the next handhold. Then I remembered something I had learned at a Body & Soul Fitness workshop. Each of our muscles has this little thing called a plus. The plus happens when you reach out your arm or leg (or whatever part) as far as you can, and then when it's at its fullest extension from the joint or point of connection, you extend it just a little more—that's the plus! One more time I reached up, but this time I gave it the plus, and it happened! I was able to reach the next handhold and pull myself up and keep going! I experienced what I call the power of the plus. We all have it in us. The power of the plus causes us to be victorious and to believe in and act on what God says is true about us.

In that moment, I realized (again) the importance and power of stretching both in our spiritual lives and in our physical lives. The Lord will often place us in situations in which He is stretching our ability to trust Him. When we turn to Him during trying times, we'll not only experience His presence, but we'll also find out that God is more than able to provide for us in any situation. The apostle Paul felt God stretching him throughout his Christian life. In fact, you might even call Paul the Flexible Apostle. Listen to how he described his life and ability to trust God in a letter he wrote to his friends in Philippi:

I have learned to be content whatever the circumstances. I know what it is to be in need, and I know what it is to have plenty. I have learned the secret of being content in any and every situation, whether well fed or hungry, whether living in plenty or in want. I can do all things through him who gives me strength (Phil. 4:11-13).

Paul flexed with whatever situation the Lord brought into his life. The Lord would stretch him and instead of depending on himself, Paul would turn to the only One who could carry the situation. With every new situation, Paul's relationship with the Lord grew closer and he could do more, knowing that the Lord would take care of him. His strength in Christ grew because he was stretched.

The same is true in our physical bodies as we stretch and take time to develop our flexibility. This final component of a wellness program is often the most neglected part of fitness, yet it can have the greatest long-term impact on your overall health and wellbeing.

To Stretch or Not to Stretch

When people are considering a new workout and how to achieve their weight-loss goals, stretching is not usually their first thought. Everyone thinks cardio first. After all, cardio plays the biggest role in increasing our metabolism and burning calories. Strength training comes second. Over the years, I've learned with just a little education and encouragement, most people see the value of lifting weights, or strength training. Once they begin to see and feel the results of strength training, they become hooked. But stretching? It's hard to see any immediate results, and it does not impact weight loss. It's not unusual for people to work with great intensity during a workout only to leave quickly at the end, without stretching, because they simply don't take the time. That's true especially for younger people, whose muscles respond quickly. But as we age, we begin to see the benefits of stretching and flexibility training.

Part of the challenge of placing an emphasis on stretching and flexibility is that the experts in the fitness field don't all agree on how important or necessary they are. The fitness field continues to do research on the validity of the two. Some experts say that stretching and flexibility training are a waste of time and make no difference in body mechanics. Others feel strongly that it is a vital part of fitness. From my experience, both personally and as a fitness instructor, I've seen firsthand the tremendous benefits of stretching.

Benefits of Stretching

In your enthusiasm to start working out, you may be tempted to skip the stretch, thinking that it is a nice thing to do but really not necessary. But the fact is that stretching warms up your muscles, lengthens them and gets them ready for action. You will run faster, throw better, jump higher, sit taller and feel better with a good stretch.[1] Consider some of the benefits of stretching in your overall fitness plan:

- *Stretching promotes and maintains range of motion in joints and improves posture.* When the muscles in the lower back are tight, it's hard to even stand up straight. When a muscle is lengthened through stretching, it exerts a greater torque on a joint to help you excel while you exercise. You'll be amazed at how a couple of minutes of stretching your back will improve your overall workout (and prevent injury).

- *Stretching offsets age-related stiffness.* Let's face it: As we age it becomes harder to move. I cannot sit in one position as long as I could when I was younger. After just 15 minutes of sitting at my computer, my legs start to stiffen up. Flexibility is primarily tied to your genetics, gender, age and level of physical activity, and some people are naturally more flexible than others.[2] However, as we age, we all lose some of our flexibility, and we may lose some range of motion in our joints. Most loss, though, is a result of inactivity rather than aging. The less active we are, the less flexible we are likely to be.[3]

- *Stretching enhances physical and mental relaxation.* Stretching not only helps to release your muscle tension but also gives you time to clear your mind as you transition into your workday. Relaxation is a state in which we experience a calm mind and a tension-free body, and it is essential to our health and wellbeing. Most of the time we are wound up so tight that we think tension is the normal state of our existence. Intentional relaxation of our muscles, however, gives us a sense of wellbeing. When we make a conscious effort to relax through techniques such as stretching accompanied by reflection, prayer and exercise, it helps our minds become calm and our bodies to become loose. In addition, a relaxed state lowers blood pressure, reduces arteriosclerosis (thickening of the arterial walls), slows down brain-cell deterioration and slows age-related memory loss.

Stretch for Success

Before stretching, take a few minutes to warm up in order to prevent injuries to your cold muscles. Begin with a simple, low-intensity warm-up such as walking while swinging the arms in a wide circle. Spend at least 5 to 10 minutes warming up prior to stretching.

F.I.T.T. Formula for Stretching

As with each part of your personal exercise program, we'll apply the F.I.T.T. formula to help you determine the best stretching routine.

- *Frequency:* Every day. Because stretching does not take much time at all and does not exhaust any muscle group, it can be done every day. Stretching should also be done before and after each workout.

- *Intensity:* Gentle stretching to the point of tension but never to the point of pain.

- *Time:* 10 to 15 minutes (to stretch all major muscle groups), holding each stretch 10 to 30 seconds. Start at the top of your body and work your way down to your feet.

- *Type:* General stretches that involve each major muscle group and connective tissue (tendon).

Guidelines to Avoid Injury

If you want to maximize each stretch and avoid painful injuries, follow these simple guidelines:

- Start each stretch slowly, exhaling as you gently stretch the muscle and inhaling as you release the stretch.
- Don't bounce a stretch. This is called "ballistic stretch." It can be effective for some elite athletes, but static stretching (gradual extension) is much gentler on the muscle groups. Bouncing gives you a longer stretch but can tear muscles. Holding a stretch while at rest is more effective and carries less risk of injury.
- Don't stretch a muscle that is not warmed up.
- Don't strain or push a muscle too far. If a stretch hurts, ease up.
- Don't hold your breath during the stretch.

Scheduling Time for Stretching

Time constraints keep many people from stretching. Some people complain that they just don't have time to stretch, while others hurry out of their fitness classes before the cool-down flexibility exercises are completed.

Ideally, taking a few minutes every day to stretch your major muscle groups will give you the most benefit. Even five minutes of stretching at the end of an exercise session is better than nothing at all. And all cardio-respiratory exercises should be followed by at least a few minutes of stretching. If you work at a sedentary job, taking a five-minute stretch break can help fight fatigue and guard against muscle strain in the lower back, neck and chest. Sitting all day can also shorten the hamstring muscles on the back of the leg, so just the simple act of standing and bending at the waist can get the blood flowing back into the legs and calves. With a bit of creative thinking, you *can* find time to stretch. Consider the following suggestions:

- If you don't have time to sufficiently warm up before stretching, try doing a few stretches immediately after a hot shower or while soaking in a hot tub. Muscles become more pliable after the hot water warms them up, and they become more receptive to stretching.

- Before getting out of bed in the morning, do a few simple stretches. Wake yourself up with a few full-body stretches by pointing your toes and reaching your arms above your head. This can clear your mind and help jump-start your morning.

- Enroll in a fitness class that concentrates on stretching. Joining a class will help you get in the habit of stretching regularly. A few fitness programs, such as Pilates and martial arts' classes, include flexibility exercises as part of their routines.

Even though stretching is such a simple thing to do, we still have a tendency to want to skip it because we think it's not important. But it *is* important: It warms up your muscles, lengthens them and gets them ready for action. Everything you do you will do better if you incorporate flexibility and stretching exercises into your daily routine.

Being Stretched by God

Walking by faith day by day, minute by minute, is certainly a vigorous exercise for many of us! Just as we need to stretch when we walk and do other exercises, we need to let God stretch us. This, too, is a vital part of our wellness program. Allowing God to stretch us lengthens our capabilities as well as our faith. One way God stretches us is when we get up in the morning for our quiet time or our exercise commitment when we don't feel like it.

In the Bible, there are many examples of common, ordinary people accomplishing amazing things when they allowed God to stretch their faith. Stretching also seemed to be one of the primary ways Jesus taught His disciples to learn to trust God for things that seem impossible.

Jesus Stretched the Disciples

One of my favorite stories of Jesus stretching His disciples appears in all four Gospels (so it must have been important!) and gives us insight into the way the Lord takes our faith to new heights.

After watching Jesus heal, preach and show compassion to those in need, it was time for the disciples to try to do these things on their own. Jesus called the 12 disciples together, divided them into pairs and gave them authority to heal and cast out evil spirits. Can you imagine that? Sure, Jesus performed these miracles, but regular, everyday fishermen and tax collectors? As Jesus sent them on their way, He gave them these instructions:

> Take nothing for the journey except a staff—no bread, no bag, no money in your belts. Wear sandals but not an extra tunic. Whenever you enter a house, stay there until you leave that town. And if any place will not welcome you or listen to you, shake the dust off your feet when you leave, as a testimony against them (Mark 6:8-11).

Now, if I had been one of Jesus' disciples at the time, I probably would have thought that He had lost His mind. *Me? Do what Jesus has been doing? No money? No food? No extra clothing?* I suspect I would have been afraid but also intrigued to try it out (much like me trying to climb a wall). The disciples went out, and they "drove out many demons and anointed many sick people with oil and healed them" (Mark 6:13). The disciples were successful and were excited at the power of God.

Now, maybe you are thinking that this is the stretching experience I was talking about, but it's not. In fact, it was when the disciples got back from their journey that Jesus stretched them. When the disciples returned to Jesus, they were amazed at how God had worked through them, but they were also really tired. Because so many people had needed help, they found that they did not even have time to eat. (I certainly know that feeling, don't you? Working from the early morning into the late evening, sometimes it's hard to find time to take care of your own needs.) Jesus, knowing that His disciples needed a break, took them away from the crowd to a quiet place to rest and regroup.

Just as they arrived, the crowds also arrived. When people are in need, they'll do whatever it takes to get help. And Jesus, having a heart of compassion, saw these lost sheep and began to teach and minister to them. As the day progressed into evening, the disciples (who were already exhausted and just wanted to be alone) asked Jesus to send the crowds away, so they could eat and have that quiet time alone. But as it so often happens in our own lives, it was at that moment when the disciples had nothing left that the Lord opened their eyes to the impossible.

Jesus could have agreed to send the crowd home. After all, the compassionate thing for His disciples would have been to let them rest. But instead, Jesus decided that stretching was the order of the day, so He told His disciples to feed the crowd. Listen in on their conversation:

But [Jesus] answered, "You give them something to eat."
They said to him, "That would take eight months of a

man's wages! Are we to go and spend that much on bread and give it to them to eat?" "How many loaves do you have?" he asked, "Go and see" (Mark 6:37-38).

More than 5,000 people had gathered, and Jesus wanted the disciples to feed them. Talk about a stretch! The disciples could not understand how what Jesus wanted could happen. But, as they would learn, all things are possible with God.

The disciples found five loaves of bread and two fish—certainly not enough to feed so many hungry people. Jesus had the disciples sit the crowd down, blessed the food that was available, and told the disciples to distribute it. With every piece of bread they handed out, their hamstrings of faith began to feel the stretch. With every fish they handed out, they were better able see life from God's perspective. Everyone was fed, plus there was plenty of food left over!

Jesus Wants to Stretch You

Do you want the rest of your life to be the best of your life? If so, allow the Lord to stretch you. How do you do that? Let's consider three quick lessons the disciples learned when Jesus fed the 5,000:

1. *They were in a place to hear the words of Jesus.* The disciples could be stretched because they took time to listen to Jesus. The first step in stretching is to make yourself available to hear God. Praying and digging into Scripture every day is the way to put yourself in position to be stretched.

2. *They acted with obedience without understanding how the problem would be solved.* The disciples were incredulous at Jesus' commands, but they still did what He said. Obeying and taking the first step of faith is often the hardest. The Lord will give you baby steps toward a goal, and you simply need to say yes to those steps and wait for further instruction. He will literally guide you along the way.

3. *They together met the needs of those in front of them.* What a powerful image: The disciples not only went out in pairs

to heal but also as a group fed the 5,000. Rarely will God call you to face an impossible situation alone. Most often, He places people to walk alongside you as you discover His plan for your life.

Stretching also comes when we realize that our gifts—our talents—are not for ourselves but for others. God wants us to take a huge leap of faith to use those gifts. Such is the case with Cris Engan. Cris is a precious First Place 4 Health leader in Brookings, South Dakota. God has been using her in a mighty way to lead others to wellness. From her story, you'll learn how God is stretching her to accomplish the even greater plans He has for her.

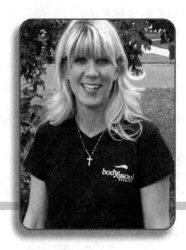

CRIS ENGAN

It is amazing how God works when you allow Him to work in you. Years have passed since I first entertained the idea of becoming an exercise instructor. I could always find a reason not to pursue the training and would decide it was not for me.

In September 2010, our church hosted a Hope 4 You event with First Place 4 Health, with Vicki herself leading an early morning boot camp. The information for Body & Soul was in the information packet for the event, and a seed buried years ago was watered! God was telling me this is something He wanted me to do. After the event, I put the papers away. Several weeks later, I came across the paper and decided to check out the website. Again I felt a strong nudge from God and ended up chatting with Vicki and others from Body & Soul. This was a stretch for me; I had been so comfortable teaching children's ministries and leading a First Place 4 Health class during the week. My familiar routine was comforting!

Besides, I thought, this exercise thing takes some talent, and I was the cheerleader who always stood in the back because she could never remember the routine. I began the journey with Body & Soul training for cardio and strength, only to find that when I was instructed to kick, my body wanted to jump; and when I was supposed to snap, I wanted to clap. Feeling defeated and unable to learn, I began to question my role in Body & Soul. Satan began to tell me that I was crazy and could not do this.

However, God is greater and more powerful, and He placed encouraging sisters in Christ in my path. Perhaps the cardio and strength was not the place for me, but boot camp is! I trust God and am willing to be used by Him, and He will show me what to do and how to do it. It is not my intent to have classes led by me; it is my intent to lead classes led by God! I enjoy how my body feels after a workout, and I also enjoy how God has used opportunities in my life to make me better able to serve Him and bring others to Christ! Sometimes the stretching is uncomfortable, but the change that occurs is a great reward. Praise be to God!

I don't mean to say that I have already achieved these things or that I have already reached perfection! But I keep working toward that day when I will finally be all that Christ Jesus saved me for and wants me to be. No, dear brothers and sisters, I am still not all I should be, but I am focusing all my energies on this one thing: Forgetting the past and looking forward to what lies ahead, I strain to reach the end of the race and receive the prize for which God, through Christ Jesus, is calling me up to heaven (see Phil. 3:12-14).

Encouragement to Stretch

Stretching arouses us to action and increases our capabilities. God has had to really stretch me over the years, especially during the hard times. I have walked through days I never thought possible. God is stretching my faith right now by providing for us financially.

We are trying to buy a house and our last child is headed off to college. What a stretch!

Consider these powerful words of Scripture that will encourage you to trust the Lord in all situations in your life:

God . . . gives life to the dead and calls things that are not as though they were (Rom. 4:17).

In other words, it is God who can bring into existence that which does not exist. For example, I did not think I had it in me to write a book, but God has stretched my capabilities, my imagination and my vocabulary. This book would not exist if He had not brought it into existence.

In 1 Timothy 1:12, Paul proclaims, "I thank Christ Jesus our Lord, who has given me strength, that he considered me faithful, appointing me to his service." God will stretch you and lengthen you to meet His criteria. He will make you equal to the task He has for you. However, He has to be the one to do it.

In Romans 8:37, Paul announces, "In all these we are more than conquerors." It's in the stretch that the power comes. Without the stretch, there is no power. Oswald Chambers, in his devotional book *My Utmost for His Highest,* says the following:

A saint's life is in the hands of God like a bow and arrow in the hands of an archer. God is aiming at something that the saint cannot see, and He stretches and strains, and every now and again the saint says—"I cannot stand any more." Yet God does not heed, He goes on stretching till His purpose is in sight, and then He lets fly. Trust yourself in God's hands.[4]

You will need to become courageous. You will need to be stout, alert, bold, solid, firm and persistent. You will need to have extreme faith to let God stretch you. Placing your faith in God is not a sign of weakness; it is a strong and valiant confidence built on your knowledge of God's love for you.

13

A Personal Wellness Plan

Carol Kent is extraordinary. Exhibiting a profoundly deep faith, an amazing amount of energy and an ability to speak in a way that makes you laugh, cry and feel loved all within the same 20 minutes, Carol is a mom with a profound sense of calling to care for her son who has been incarcerated for over 11 years.

If anyone has a strong sense of God's ability to provide, Carol is the woman. With her busy schedule, Carol struggled to exercise and stick to an eating plan that would help her to live a long healthy life. A few years ago, Carol asked me to help her develop a wellness plan that she could stick to, so we met and I asked my usual series of questions to determine what would motivate her to follow a wellness program for a lifetime. Here's an excerpt of my interview with Carol:

Vicki: Carol, tell me a little bit about your life and what has been keeping you from focusing on your health.

Carol: I am a writer and speaker, and life is busy. I travel three to four days a week in out-of-state ministry, sometimes arriving for a speaking engagement just in time to change my clothes and get to the venue. I usually stay in hotels or conference centers on these trips, and I'm often at a banquet or retreat where the meals are all alike (usually with dessert), or I'm being taken to the meeting planner's favorite restaurant. Plates filled with caloric meals face me everywhere I go, so discipline (eating less than is on the plate) is a tough decision. Also, I do not have the luxury of big chunks of time for exercise when I'm away from home, and I have rationalized that I'm preparing for ministry or I'm winding down after ministry. It is a good excuse for not doing it.

Vicki: So from what you are telling me, you're tired of making excuses for not exercising. Do you think you've believed any lies about yourself, wellness or God's love for you?

Carol: Without verbalizing it, I believed the lie that ministry is more important than physical exercise. Both are important, but without physical exercise, the ministry I'm called to do will be energy depleting and overwhelmingly exhausting. I know what I need to do: Stop making excuses and start making the right choices.

Vicki: Is there a specific excuse you need to get rid of?

Carol: Yes, that I don't have time to exercise. We all make time for what we really want to do, and I never wanted to exercise enough to make it a part of my day-to-day life. If I wear clothes that cover a little excess weight, I rationalize that the 20 extra pounds didn't really matter.

Vicki: What benefit of exercise do you need most in your life?

Carol: I need more energy and stamina, and I need more time on this earth. I work at my favorite hobby, which is ministry that includes evangelism; equipping Christians to communicate effectively; speaking at conferences, retreats and arena events on Bible-based themes; along with writing books based on God's truth. I would like to be actively involved in His kingdom agenda for many years to come. Also, my husband has asked me on numerous occasions to do daily exercise with him, because he is well aware that the quality of our future years will be directly proportional to how active we continue to be and on the quality of our diet.

Vicki: Those are great benefits to focus on. Now tell me, what is going to motivate you to keep you going when it gets tough?

Carol: Needing to live as long as I can! I don't know if you know about our son, JP. He is serving a life sentence in a state prison in Florida for first-degree murder. He has no chance of ever getting out on parole. Every Sunday that we are not involved in ministry, my husband, Gene, and I visit him. He is our only child. I have a large and loving family, and they are very supportive. But my husband and I are the only ones who regularly visit JP, because our family members live out-of-state. I need to live as long as I can to be an advocate for my son, to encourage him when he is lonely; and to be a strong, spiritual support to the ministry he has behind the razor wire of a maximum security prison. I sometimes wonder, *When my husband and I are gone, who will visit our son?* That's strong motivation for needing to stay healthy for as long as possible.

Vicki: Have you found a verse in the Bible that you can cling to and that will speak truth into your life and that will keep you going?

Carol: Yes, Isaiah 43:19 has provided tremendous encouragement to me: "See, I am doing a new thing! Now it springs up; do you not perceive it? I am making a way in the desert and streams in the wasteland."

Vicki: Perfect. Let's write the plan.

Carol and I worked through her Get Fit Plan that you'll find at the end of this chapter. As I prepared for this book, I emailed Carol and asked her what has happened since that first interview. Here's what she wrote.

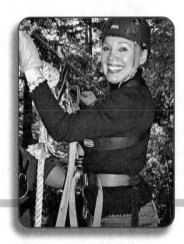

CAROL KENT

Over the last year, on our at-home days, Gene and I began walking four miles a day. (If you do 15-minute miles, it takes an hour.) During our ministry trips, on one or two of the days we were away from home, we walked for an hour on a treadmill at our hotel or outside when weather permitted. Sometimes flight schedules and ministry commitments kept us from our goal one or two days a week, but we got back on track once back home.

We started eating only one bite of dessert, instead of finishing it off when we were at events where preplanned meals were served. We made our at-home days our more restricted diet days and learned the many creative ways you can build a salad with fresh vegetables, salmon or chicken, and we enjoyed our meals! Two exciting things happened:

1. We have both lost more than 20 pounds over the past year.
2. Our four-mile-a-day walks have become special times of bonding as a couple, and we began prayer walking during a part of each of those hours, praying for the needs of our son and people we know. That has truly been transformational!

Thanks, Vicki, for motivating me to get started and helping me form an action-plan that still works today!

What I've done with Carol and many other people around the country, I would like to do with you. Over the next few pages, we are going to talk honestly about your life, your motivations, the lies you've believed and the excuses you've made. Consider this your personal interview and call to action.

Let's Talk

The time you and I spend together is vitally important for your success. It will be the final piece of my involvement with you and the development of your wellness plan. The rest will be up to you. This first step will be one of self-examination. You may have all of the knowledge and understanding that you need but just have not been able to turn it into action. Are you ready? I'm going to push you a little, so get ready.

First, let's pray together:

Lord Jesus, thank You for the opportunity to work with another one of Your special and precious children. Thank You for Your deep love for each of us and Your desire for us to live a life of joy, strength and hope. May Your Holy Spirit guide and direct this conversation as we pursue our best. In Jesus' name, amen.

All right, so tell me, how is your relationship with the Lord today? Are you walking close to God? Are there areas in your life that you don't want the Lord to see? Are you walking in obedience in each area of your life?

Over the years, I have found that most people have areas in their life that they prefer not to address with the Lord. When we have unconfessed sin in our lives, however, it creates a barrier to fully experiencing the fullness of God's love and blessing. In order to start a wellness plan that will transform us, we need to get brutally honest with the Lord. A vital component of success is our willingness to do what God commands us to do. Obedience brings blessings and peace; disobedience brings fear and breeds more disobedience.

I've learned the hard way about obedience. I work hard at maintaining my spiritual life in addition to my physical fitness, because they are intimately connected. I am constantly amazed at how confessing sin, experiencing God's forgiveness and then choosing to live as God has called me impact my desire and ability to live as fully and abundantly as God wants me to live. The same will be true for you.

The Lord's Plan for Blessing

Thousands of years ago, the Lord developed His own Get Fit plan for the people of Israel. After laying out the Ten Commandments, the Lord set out a plan for His people to experience great blessings for obedience as described in Deuteronomy 28:1-14. This part of the Old Testament is a joy to read! Here are just some of the blessings that are listed:

- Blessed in the city and the country (v. 3)
- Blessed by the fruit of your womb (v. 4)
- Blessed in your crops (v. 4)
- Blessed in your herds (v. 4)
- Blessed in your basket and kneading trough (v. 5)
- Blessed when you come in and blessed when you go out (v. 6)

Wow! All of this is promised to those who are obedient to the Lord our God. When I read about the possibility for a blessed life, I am motivated to follow God's plan. And I am obedient . . . well, most days. When I studied God's plan in this chapter of Deuteronomy, I found the Holy Spirit leading me away from the word "blessed," highlighting instead words like "fully obey" and "carefully follow" (v. 1). God called me to notice the small things in His plans, and when I did that, I could see the possibility of being obedient in the *big* things.

Attention to the Small Things

When I pay attention to the small things in my life and make sure they line up with God's will and purpose for me, I am truly blessed in just about everything I do! This is exactly what He promises in

His Word. When I walk with the Lord, my life is full of peace and I am assured of God's love for me. Just the opposite happens when I am not careful. There have been times in the past that I have not been careful and I have disobeyed God. I always have good excuses, but they are still just excuses.

This is the truth: God wants our full obedience and full attention to the small details of our lives. The Bible tells us that if we are faithful in the small things, He will bless us with big things! When I am walking with God in obedience, His peace and presence in my life are beautiful things!

Here is an example of how my success is dependent on obedience: God has told me through His Word and through His Holy Spirit that for me to remain faithful to my wellness goals, I must keep track of my life. A passage of Scripture that has helped me in this area is John 15:9-11:

> As the Father has loved me, so have I loved you. Now remain in my love. If you obey my commands, you will remain in my love, just as I have obeyed my Father's commands and remain in his love. I have told you this so that my joy may be in you and that your joy may be complete.

This Scripture very clearly says that God wants to bless my life and wants it to be full of *joy*. It's His job to bless me, and it's my job to be obedient. The whole of my life needs to demonstrate my close relationship with God. This means spending time with the Lord, loving all the people He places in my path, and being a good caretaker of His most personal gifts to me: my body, mind and spirit.

Over the years, I've found that it's not the big temptations that trip me up in my weight-loss goals; it's the small things. Instead of worrying about how much weight I need to lose, I need to eat right, one meal at a time, and exercise consistently, one day at a time. When I do those things, I will reach my goals. When I focus on a weight-loss goal or food I'm giving up, I easily get distracted.

A Journal for the Record

The best way to stay obedient in the small and daily work of getting in shape is to keep a journal. I record what I eat and how much I exercise. The act of writing the information down helps me to celebrate small successes and to notice if I'm starting to slip. When I am obedient in this small thing, God blesses me. As a direct result of my disobedience in this small thing, my priorities fall out of order and I struggle to keep my wellness commitments. I become fearful and doubt His word; I believe the lies and am tempted to quit! That is not what God wants for me. Disobedience robs me of joy, replacing it with fear!

Confession Is Good for the Soul (and Body!)

Wellness is more about progress than perfection. In fact, if you are going for perfection, you'll quickly get discouraged and quit. However, if you see your life as a series of successes and slip-ups, you'll be able to move forward toward your goals. When you move away from your goals, it's time to simply get back on track by following these simple steps:

1. *Confess.* Identify what it is you have not been willing to tell the Lord about where you are failing. Truth sets you free, literally. When you honestly talk with the Lord, you'll feel better right away. You may be embarrassed, but He already knows the truth. He's just waiting for you to tell it to Him.

2. *Ask for forgiveness.* God loves you, and His greatest desire is for you to live a holy life that is filled with His joy. He loved you so much that He sent His Son to die so that you might be forgiven. All you need to do is ask Him for forgiveness.

3. *Embrace God's love.* The Lord has forgiven you, but it's up to you to accept His gift. One of the saddest mo-

ments I have experienced in working with others is when someone believes in God's forgiveness in his or her mind but doesn't receive it in his or her heart. When you receive God's love, you'll feel both empowered and excited to serve Him.

Sin that is not dealt with has the potential to wreck your progress. It is a huge obstacle to the work of the Holy Spirit. He is already at work in us, but we need to cooperate! It is always a good idea to start with a fresh, clean slate, so deal with your sin whenever you sin.

Your Fitness Plan

Are you ready to develop your personal plan to Get Fit? Before you fill out the chart, let me tell you about the questions you need to ask yourself and things that you need to think about.

What Lie Do I Need to Stop Believing?

Is there a lie you have believed about yourself that you know now is untrue? Identify the lie and write it down. In a recent consultation when I asked this question, the response was "I have believed that I am lazy and I know that I am not lazy. That is a lie that I know in my heart is not true."

What Is the Truth I Need to Focus On?

For every lie you believe about yourself, the Lord wants to give you His truth. If you believe that you are lazy, the truth you'll need to embrace is that God made you to work hard and has given you the resources you need to do the work He has called you to do. Even in your weakness, He will be strong.

But he said to me, "My grace is sufficient for you, for my power is made perfect in weakness." Therefore I will boast all the more gladly about my weakness, so that Christ's power may rest on me (2 Cor. 12:9).

In your times of prayer and Bible study, the Lord will show you what truth He has for you.

What Excuse Do I Need to Get Rid Of?

There is a reason that you have not been doing what you know you need to do. What is it? Perhaps, like Carol, your excuse is that you don't have the time. After reading chapter 2 ("Lies that Steal, Kill and Destroy"), do you still want to hold on to that excuse? Whatever excuse you are holding on to, allow the Holy Spirit to give you a new vision of yourself, and throw that excuse out!

One way to find out what excuse has become your obstacle is to ask your family or close friends what words you use to describe yourself when talking about getting in shape. You'll be surprised at how they can use your words to help you find which excuse you need to identify. You need brutal honesty, so ask them to tell you in love, and have fun—humor sometimes helps to identify your excuses.

What Benefit of Exercise Do I Need to Focus On?

So, what will a new and healthy you look like one year from now? What will you be able to do that you cannot do now? Will there be a mission trip you will have the energy for? Will you be able to lower your insurance rates by saving money when you come off medications? Will your knees stop hurting from so much pressure? Will you be able to sleep better? Will you handle stress better?

What Motivation Will Sustain Me?

Review the benefits you've read about. Which ones have appealed to you? Have you identified with any of the testimonies you've read in these pages? Dream realistically from God's perspective: How does the Lord want to bless you in your obedience? The strongest motivator of all is love, and the motivation with eternal value will keep you going the longest. So what will keep you going? When you are a fit and healthy person, what contribution to the Kingdom will you be able to make? In whose life do you want to have an eternal influence?

What Scripture Verse Will Be My Fitness Verse?

In the appendix of this book is a list of Scripture memory verses. The Bible is full of wonderful truths that will set you free and empower you to live beyond your current circumstances. Search the Scriptures for yourself or read through the verses in the appendix. Choose a verse, memorize it, and treasure it. God's Word will bring you life.

When the Lord shows you what truth He wants you to focus on, that truth may become your fitness verse. I have often seen the Lord give a specific verse to a person who is honest about himself or herself. That verse can become a tool that God uses to keep you motivated.

Have I Realized that Wellness Is an Act of Worship?

Finally, have you come to the realization that your wellness journey can be an act of worship as you present your body to God daily? The disciplines you will need to follow in order to reach your goals will involve some of the hardest work you have ever done, but knowing that you are doing it as a sacrifice to Him will make all of the difference.

Do I Have a Witness?

As your first act of commitment, I want you to sign and date the fitness plan and have someone witness it. If we were sitting down together, I would go over each of these questions with you, formulate the plan and be your witness. It's important to share publically the commitments you make privately. You do not have to announce it in church on Sunday morning, but asking one person whom you trust to sign as your witness will hold you accountable and help you be sober minded about your plan.

Remember my interview with Carol Kent? I had her fill out this form in response to the questions. Here's what she wrote:

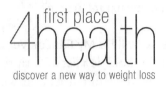

MY GET FIT PLAN

Stop believing the lies.

- Focus on the truth.
- Get rid of excuses.
- Focus on the benefits of exercise and not my pain.
- Identify a sustaining motivation for my wellness endeavors.
- Find my fitness verse.
- Consider my wellness endeavors an act of worship.

Heart Work

What lie do I need to stop believing?

At this time there is no lie I am believing; just excuses!

What is the truth I need to focus on?

That God will help me in my wellness endeavors because He cares for me.

What excuse do I need to get rid of?

That I do not have time to exercise.

What benefit of exercise do I need to focus on?

Energy and longevity.

My sustaining motivation:

To be there for JP as long as possible.

My Fitness Verse
Isaiah 43:19: "See, I am doing a new thing! Now it springs up; do you not perceive it? I am making a way in the desert and streams in the wasteland."

Steps to Fitness
Steps I can take to improve my fitness levels:

- Cardiovascular:

  Frequency: _5x a week_
  Intensity: _Moderate_
  Time: _30 minutes_
  Type: _Walking_

- Strength Training:

  Frequency: _2x a week_
  Intensity: _5 lbs weights_
  Time: _15 min_
  Type: _DVD workout_

- Stretching and Flexibility:

  Frequency: _Every day_
  Intensity: _Gentle_
  Time: _10 minutes_
  Type: _DVD_

- BMI: _I will eat 1,500 calories a day, and record my food in my food journal daily._

I commit to carry out these wellness endeavors as an act of worship for my Lord and Savior Jesus Christ, for my good and His glory.

Name: _Carol Kent_ Date: _____ Witness: _Vicki Heath_

Now it's your turn. I would like you to thoughtfully and prayerfully consider the questions on the form on the following pages and fill in the blanks. Take all of the time you need and be honest. Your answers are the keys to your lifetime of wellness.

The Journey Begins

Do you remember as a child getting ready for a family trip? Whether it was a day trip to the beach or an extended vacation across the country, you (or your parents) needed to make plans and get things ready.

Do you remember the feeling of sitting in the car after all the plans were made and you were ready to pull out of the driveway? Imagine if after planning and packing for a great adventure you got into the car and just sat there worrying that maybe it just wasn't worth going on the trip after all. Imagine, if after all that work, you decided it just wasn't the right time to go on an adventure.

The only way to experience the benefits of the journey is to start it. And the time for that start is now. Get excited about how the Lord is going to use this next season in your life to bless you. I'm already excited for you!

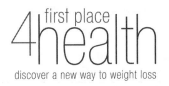

MY GET FIT PLAN

Stop believing the lies.

- Focus on the truth.
- Get rid of excuses.
- Focus on the benefits of exercise and not my pain.
- Identify a sustaining motivation for my wellness endeavors.
- Find my fitness verse.
- Consider my wellness endeavors an act of worship.

Heart Work
What lie do I need to stop believing?

_____

_____

_____

_____

What is the truth I need to focus on?

_____

_____

_____

_____

What excuse do I need to get rid of?

_____

_____

_____

My sustaining motivation:

_____

_____

My Fitness Verse

_____

_____

Steps to Fitness

Steps I can take to improve my fitness levels:

- Cardiovascular:

    Frequency: _____
    Intensity: _____
    Time: _____
    Type: _____

- Strength Training:

    Frequency: _____
    Intensity: _____
    Time: _____
    Type: _____

- Stretching and Flexibility:

    Frequency: _____
    Intensity: _____
    Time: _____
    Type: _____

- BMI: _____

I commit to carry out these wellness endeavors as an act of worship for my Lord and Savior Jesus Christ, for my good and His glory.

Name: _____ Date: _____ Witness: _____

Living in the Zone

Living in the zone—*finally!* If someone walked up to you and asked, "What does it mean to play in the zone?" how would you respond? Does a professional athlete come to mind when you think of being *in the zone*? You don't have to be an athlete to understand what "living in the zone" means, because now you have all that you need to live there for the rest of your life!

To live in the zone means you are unstoppable, successful and consistent. You are operating totally in God's strength. Your weaknesses are no longer causing you failure, because God is changing them into strengths. You are running the race called life with the mind of Christ.

The 1924 Olympic runner Eric Liddell once said, "God made me fast. When I run, I feel God's pleasure. To win is to glorify Him." You too can please and glorify God by staying in the zone. You will feel God's pleasure as you work to follow your fitness plan. You will run your own race to achieve your wellness goals (even if the achievements are small ones), and when you do, you will glorify God.

Let's review. There are some simple things we can do to stay in the zone:

- Run your own race.
- Realize and appreciate your uniqueness.
- Learn to take a hit.

Champions don't compare themselves to others, and they don't run somebody else's race. They seek out the competition and are exhilarated by each hit they may have to take because they know it leads to victory along the way. Champions overcome and

learn from past failures and persevere beyond the obstacles life
throws at them.

I pray that you, my dear friends, will know your weaknesses,
trust God for your strengths and move beyond your self-imposed
limitations to the true heart and spirit of the champions God intends for you to be!

Run your own race, and live life in the zone!

Prayer of the Champion

Lord, my goal is to live in such a way as to leave behind
Your mark and not my own. It is hard. I get tired and sometimes
I am consumed with my life. Lord, break the hold that this world
and its cares have on me. My prayer is that everyone who You
put in my path will know that it is all about You and that You
alone lead us in the way everlasting!

APPENDIX

Scripture Memory Verses

I am giving you this list of Scripture verses as a starting point. You will discover that the Bible provides encouragement for every area of life in which you may struggle. Unfortunately, I can guarantee that there will definitely be days you will struggle on your wellness journey. You will face difficult circumstances; you will be tempted to give up; you will need guidance in making good choices; and you will continually need the Holy Spirit to teach you the truth.

God's Word can help you overcome every reason or excuse you can come up with for not getting fit. Excuses will continue to creep back into your mind if you are not careful. But when God's Word becomes firmly rooted in your mind, not only will your thoughts connect with God's thoughts, but you also will experience His power as never before. Scripture memorization and meditation will make a permanent change in your thought patterns. God's Word will be food for you, bringing life to your bones and joy to your heart.

Finding Hope

Psalm 40:1-3: "I waited patiently for the LORD; he turned to me and heard my cry. He lifted me out of the slimy pit, out of the mud and mire; he set my feet on a rock and gave me a firm place to stand. He put a new song in my mouth, a hymn of praise to our God. Many will see and fear and put their trust in the LORD."

Psalm 40:4: "Blessed is the man who makes the LORD his trust, who does not look to the proud, to those who turn aside to false gods."

Psalm 69:1-2: "Save me, O God, for the waters have come up to my neck. I sink in the miry depths where there is no foothold."

Psalm 139:13-16: "You created my inmost being; you knit me to-gether in my mother's womb. I praise you because I am fearfully and wonderfully made; your works are wonderful, I know that full well. My frame was not hidden from you when I was made in the secret place. When I was woven together in the depths of the earth, your eyes saw my unformed body. All the days ordained for me were writ-ten in your book before one of them came to be."

John 16:33: "[Jesus said,] 'In this world you will have trouble. But take heart! I have overcome the world.'"

Galatians 6:2: "Carry each other's burdens, and in this way you will fulfill the law of Christ."

James 4:10: "Humble yourselves before the Lord, and he will lift you up."

Hebrews 12:1-3: "Therefore, since we are surrounded by such a great cloud of witnesses, let us throw off everything that hinders and the sin that so easily entangles, and let us run with perseverance the race marked out for us. Let us fix our eyes on Jesus, the author and perfecter of our faith, who for the joy set before him endured the cross, scorning its shame, and sat down at the right hand of the throne of God. Consider him who endured such opposition from sinful men, so that you will not grow weary and lose heart."

Handling the Truth

Psalm 37:5: "Commit your way to the LORD; trust in him and he will do this."

Psalm 89:15: "Blessed are those who have learned to acclaim you, who walk in the light of your presence, O LORD."

Proverbs 3:5-6: "Trust in the LORD with all of your heart and lean not on your own understanding; in all your ways acknowledge him, and he will make your paths straight."

John 10:10: "The thief comes only to steal and kill and destroy; I have come that they may have life, and have it to the full."

1 Corinthians 2:16: " 'For who has known the mind of the Lord that he may instruct him?' But we have the mind of Christ."

1 John 3:1: "How great is the love the Father has lavished on us, that we should be called children of God! And that is what we are!"

A New Way of Thinking

Psalm 1:1-2: "Blessed is the man who does not walk in the counsel of the wicked or stand in the way of sinners or sit in the seat of mockers. But his delight is in the law of the LORD, and on his law he meditates day and night."

Isaiah 43:19: "See, I am doing a new thing! Now it springs up; do you not perceive it? I am making a way in the desert and streams in the wasteland."

Luke 9:23: "[Jesus said,] 'If anyone would come after me, he must deny himself and take up his cross daily and follow me.' "

Romans 8:6: "The mind of sinful man is death, but the mind controlled by the Spirit is life and peace."

2 Corinthians 5:17: "If anyone is in Christ, he is a new creation; the old has gone, the new has come!"

Ephesians 3:20: "Now to him who is able to do immeasurably more than all we ask or imagine, according to his power that is at work within us."

Philippians 4:8: "Brothers, whatever is true, whatever is noble, whatever is right, whatever is pure, whatever is lovely, whatever is admirable— if anything is excellent or praiseworthy—think about such things."

Overcoming Obstacles

Psalm 90:12: "Teach us to number our days aright, that we may gain a heart of wisdom."

Psalm 118:5-7: "In my anguish I cried to the LORD, and he answered by setting me free. The LORD is with me; I will not be afraid. What can man do to me? The LORD is with me; he is my helper. I will look in triumph on my enemies."

Ecclesiastes 4:9-12: "Two are better than one, because they have a good return for their work: If one falls down, his friend can help him up. But pity the man who falls and has no one to help him up! Also, if two lie down together, they will keep warm. But how can one keep warm alone? Though one may be overpowered, two can defend themselves. A cord of three strands is not quickly broken."

Romans 12:11-12: "Never be lacking in zeal, but keep your spiritual fervor, serving the Lord. Be joyful in hope, patient in affliction, faithful in prayer."

Galatians 6:9: "Let us not become weary in doing good, for at the proper time we will reap a harvest if we do not give up."

Sustaining Motivation

Psalm 119:148: "My eyes stay open through the watches of the night, that I may meditate on your promises."

Proverbs 16:2: "All a man's ways seem innocent to him, but motives are weighed by the LORD."

Matthew 11:28-29: "Come to me all you who are weary and burdened, and I will give you rest. Take my yoke upon you and learn from me, for I am gentle and humble in heart, and you will find rest for your souls."

Matthew 22:37-40: " 'Love the Lord your God with all your heart and with all your soul and with all your mind.' This is the first and greatest commandment. And the second is like it: 'Love your neighbor as yourself.' All the Law and the Prophets hang on these two commandments."

Romans 12:3: "Do not think of yourself more highly than you ought, but rather think of yourself with sober judgment, in accordance with the measure of faith God has given you."

1 Corinthians 6:19-20: "Do you not know that your body is a temple of the Holy Spirit, who is in you, whom you have received from God? You are not your own; you were bought at a price. Therefore honor God with your body."

A New Way to Worship

Psalm 105:4: "Look to the LORD and his strength; seek his face always."

1 Chronicles 21:24: "But King David replied to Araunah, 'No, I insist on paying the full price. I will not take for the LORD what is yours, or sacrifice a burnt offering that costs me nothing.' "

John 4:23-24: "Yet a time is coming and has now come when the true worshipers will worship the Father in spirit and truth, for they are the kind of worshipers the Father seeks. God is spirit, and his worshipers must worship in spirit and in truth."

Romans 12:1: "Therefore, I urge you, brothers, in view of God's mercy, to offer your bodies as living sacrifices, holy and pleasing to God—this is your spiritual act of worship."

1 Thessalonians 5:23: "May God himself, the God of peace, sanctify you through and through. May your whole spirit, soul and body be kept blameless at the coming of our Lord Jesus Christ."

The Importance of Rest

Genesis 2:2-3: "By the seventh day God had finished the work he had been doing; so on the seventh day he rested from all his work. And God blessed the seventh day and made it holy, because on it he rested from all the work of creating that he had done."

Psalm 127:1-2: "Unless the LORD builds the house, its builders labor in vain. Unless the LORD watches over the city, the watchmen stand guard in vain. In vain you rise early and stay up late, toiling for food to eat—for he grants sleep to those he loves."

Luke 10:41-42: " 'Martha, Martha,' the Lord answered, 'you are worried and upset about many things, but only one thing is needed. Mary has chosen what is better, and it will not be taken away from her.' "

John 15:5-6: "I am the vine; you are the branches. If a man remains in me and I in him, he will bear much fruit; apart from me you can do nothing. If anyone does not remain in me, he is like a branch that is thrown away and withers; such branches are picked up, thrown into the fire and burned."

1 Peter 5:7: "Cast all your anxiety on him because he cares for you."

A New Relationship with Food

Psalm 63:5: "My soul will be satisfied as with the richest foods; with singing lips my mouth will praise you."

Proverbs 24:13-14: "Eat honey, my son, for it is good; honey from the comb is sweet to your taste. Know also that wisdom is sweet to your soul; if you find it, there is a future hope for you, and your hope will not be cut off."

Ecclesiastes 6:7: "All man's efforts are for his mouth, yet his appetite is never satisfied."

John 4:34: " 'My food,' said Jesus, 'is to do the will of him who sent me and to finish his work.' "

Romans 12:15: "Rejoice with those who rejoice; mourn with those who mourn."

Romans 14:17: "For the kingdom of God is not a matter of eating and drinking, but of righteousness, peace and joy in the Holy Spirit."

1 Peter 5:8: "Be self-controlled and alert. Your enemy the devil prowls around like a roaring lion looking for someone to devour."

The Importance of Exercise

Proverbs 17:17: "A friend loves at all times, and a brother is born for adversity."

Isaiah 40:28-31: "Do you not know? Have you not heard? The LORD is the everlasting God, the Creator of the ends of the earth. He will not grow tired or weary, and his understanding no one can fathom. He gives strength to the weary and increases the power of the weak. Even youths grow tired and weary, and young men stumble and fall; but those who hope in the LORD will renew their strength. They will soar on wings like eagles; they will run and not grow weary, they will walk and not be faint."

Philippians 3:13-14: "Brothers, I do not consider myself yet to have taken hold of it. But one thing I do: Forgetting what is behind and straining toward what is ahead, I press on toward the goal to win the prize for which God has called me heavenward in Christ Jesus."

1 Timothy 4:8: "For physical training is of some value, but godliness has value for all things, holding promise for both the present life and the life to come."

Heart Care

Proverbs 4:20-23: "My son, pay attention to what I say; listen closely to my words. Do not let them out of your sight, keep them within your heart; for they are life to those who find them and health to a man's whole body. Above all else, guard your heart, for it is the well-spring of life."

Proverbs 14:30: "A heart at peace gives life to the body, but envy rots the bones."

1 Chronicles 22:19: "Now devote your heart and soul to seeking the LORD your God."

Philippians 4:6-7: "Do not be anxious about anything, but in everything, by prayer and petition, with thanksgiving, present your requests to God. And the peace of God, which transcends all understanding, will guard your hearts and your minds in Christ Jesus."

Strength Training

Numbers 14:9: "Do not be afraid of the people of the land, because we will swallow them up. Their protection is gone, but the LORD is with us. Do not be afraid of them."

Joshua 1:6-7: "Be strong and courageous, because you will lead these people to inherit the land I swore to their forefathers to give them. Be strong and very courageous. Be careful to obey all the law my servant Moses gave you; do not turn from it to the right or to the left, that you may be successful wherever you go."

Psalm 31:24: "Be strong and take heart, all you who hope in the LORD."

Flexibility and Stretching

Isaiah 54:2: "Enlarge the place of your tent, stretch your tent curtains wide, do not hold back; lengthen your cords, strengthen your stakes."

Matthew 12:13: "Then he said to the man, 'Stretch out your hand.' So he stretched it out and it was completely restored, just as sound as the other.'"

Romans 8:35-37: "Who shall separate us from the love of Christ? Shall trouble or hardship or persecution or famine or nakedness or danger or sword? As it is written: 'For your sake we face death all day long; we are considered as sheep to be slaughtered.' No, in all these things we are more than conquerors through him who loved us."

Philippians 3:12-14: "Not that I have already obtained all this, or have already been made perfect, but I press on to take hold of that for which Christ Jesus took hold of me."

Philippians 4:11-13: "I have learned to be content whatever the circumstances. I know what it is to be in need, and I know what it is to have plenty. I have learned the secret of being content in any and every situation, whether well fed or hungry, whether living in plenty or in want. I can do all things through him who gives me strength."

1 Timothy 1:12: "I thank Christ Jesus our Lord, who has given me strength, that he considered me faithful, appointing me to his service."

A Personal Wellness Plan

Deuteronomy 28:1-2: "If you obey the LORD your God and carefully follow all his commands I give you today, the LORD your God will set you high above all the nations on the earth. All these blessings will come upon you and accompany you if you obey the LORD your God."

John 15:9-11: "As the Father has loved me, so have I loved you. Now remain in my love. If you obey my commands, you will remain in my love, just as I have obeyed my Father's commands and remain in his love. I have told you this so that my joy may be in you and that your joy may be complete."

Endnotes

Chapter 3: A New Way of Thinking
1. "Memorization of the Bible," *Parade Magazine*, February 11, 1962. http://www.ser monillustrations.com/a-z/m/memorization_of_the_bible.htm (accessed May 2011).
2. Lisa Young, *The Portion Teller: Smartsize Your Way to Permanent Weight Loss* (New York: Crown Archetype, 2005).

Chapter 4: Obstacles and Ways to Overcome Them
1. Catrine Tudor-Locke and David R. Bassett Jr., "How Many Steps/Day Are Enough?" *University of Utah College of Health*, 2004. http://www.health.utah.edu/peak/Health_ Fitness/Tudor%20Locke%20Paper.pdf (accessed May 2011).
2. Mayo Clinic Staff, "Walking: Trim Your Waistline, Improve Your Health," December 18, 2010. http://www.mayoclinic.com/health/walking/HQ01612 (accessed March 2011).
3. "Number of Daily Steps Impacts Obesity Factors in Women," American College of Sports Medicine, May 5, 2004. http://www.acsm.org/AM/Template.cfm?Section= Home_Page&template=/CM/ContentDisplay.cfm&ContentID=4214.
4. Mayo Clinic Staff, "Walking: Trim Your Waistline, Improve Your Health."

Chapter 5: Motivation for a Lifetime
1. Leslie Leyland Fields, "A Feast Fit for the King: Returning the Growing Fields and Kitchen Table to God," *Christianity Today*, November 5, 2010. http://www.christianitytoday.com /ct/2010/november/9.22.html (accessed May 2011).
2. Daisy May, "Obesity in the Christian World: Defeating Discrimination from Church Peers," *Associated Content from Yahoo!* July 19, 2005. http://www.associatedcontent.com/ article/5746/obesity_in_the_christian_world.html?cat=5 (accessed March 2011).

Chapter 6: A New Way to Worship
1. Brother Lawrence, *Practicing the Presence of God: A Modernized Christian Classic* (Brewster, MA: Paraclete Press, 2007).
2. "The Competitor's Creed," *Fellowship of Christian Athletes*, 2011. http://www.fca.org/ TEAMFCA/CompetitorsCreed.lsp (accessed May 2011).

Chapter 7: The Importance of Rest
1. G. E. Miller, "The U.S. Is the Most Overworked Developed Nation in the World—When Do We Draw the Line?" *20somethingfinance.com*, October 12, 2010. http://20something finance.com/american-hours-worked-productivity-vacation (accessed March 2011).
2. "Less Stress, More Sleep Can Help with Weight Loss: Study," *Edmonton Sun*, March 29, 2011. http://www.edmontonsun.com/life/healthandfitness/2011/03/29/17791641.html (accessed May 2011).
3. Richard B. Couey, lecture at Baylor University, Waco, Texas.
4. Michael H. Bonnet and Donna L. Arand, "How Much Sleep Do Adults Need?" *National Sleep Foundation*, 2011. http://www.sleepfoundation.org/article/white-papers/ how-much-sleep-do-adults-need (accessed April 2011).
5. "Stress May Cause Excess Abdominal Fat in Otherwise Slender Women, Study Conducted at Yale Shows," Yale University, September/October 2000. http://opac.yale.edu/news/ article.aspx?id=3386.
6. Matthew M. Burg, "Stress, Behavior, and Heart Disease," *Yale University School of Medicine Heart Book*, 1992, *Yale School of Medicine*, 2011. http://www.med.yale.edu/library/ heartbk/8.pdf (accessed March 2011).
7. Beth Moore, *Living Beyond Yourself: Exploring the Fruit of the Spirit* (Nashville, TN: Lifeway Christian Resources, 2004).
8. Ibid.

Chapter 8: A New Relationship with Food
1. Krista M. C. Cline and Kenneth F. Ferraro, "Does Religion Increase the Prevalence and Incidence of Obesity in Adulthood?" *Journal for the Scientific Study of Religion,* vol. 45, no. 2 (2006).
2. Cathleen Falsani, "Weighty Matter: Is Religion Making Us Fat?" *Chicago Sun Times,* August 26, 2006.
3. Steve Reynolds, *Bod4God: The Four Keys to Losing Weight* (Ventura, CA: Regal Books, 2009).
4. *First Place 4 Health Member's Guide* (Ventura, CA: Regal Books, 2008), p. 82.
5. Reynolds, *Bod4God,* p. 20.

Chapter 9: The Importance of Exercise
1. *First Place 4 Health Member's Guide* (Ventura, CA: Regal Books, 2008), p. 182.
2. "Obesity and Cancer: Questions and Answers," *National Cancer Institute at the National Institutes of Health,* March 16, 2004. http://www.cancer.gov/cancertopics/factsheet/Risk/obesity (accessed May 2011).
3. *First Place 4 Health Member's Guide,* p. 183.
4. Ibid.
5. Ibid.
6. Ibid.
7. Ibid.
8. Harvard School of Public Health Press Releases, "Women Who Reduce Sedentary Behaviors Significantly Reduce Risk for Type 2 Diabetes and Obesity," *Harvard School of Public Health,* 2003. http://www.hsph.harvard.edu/news/press-releases/archives/2003-releases/press04082003.html (accessed May 2011).
9. *First Place 4 Health Member's Guide,* p. 183.
10. Ibid., pp. 183-184.
11. Ibid., p. 184.
12. Ibid., citing "Exercise May Lower Risk of Colds," *The Stress of Life.com,* July 20, 2005. http://thestressoflife.com/exercise_may_lower_risk_of_colds.htm (accessed May 2011).
13. Ibid., p. 184.
14. Ibid., citing Dulce Zamora, "Eat, Exercise, Relax and Sleep Your Way to Better Sex," *MedicineNet.com,* February 2, 2005. http://www.medicinenet.com/script/main/art.asp?articlekey=55996 (accessed May 2011).
15. Charlene Laino, "Brain Exercises May Delay Memory Loss: Study Shows Activities Like Reading Magazines Are Linked to Lower Risk of Dementia," *WebMD,* April 29, 2009. http://www.webmd.com/brain/news/20090429/brain-exercises-may-delay-memory-loss (accessed May 2011).
16. *First Place 4 Health Member's Guide,* pp. 186-187.
17. Ibid., p. 113.
18. Ibid., pp. 109-111.
19. Steve Mitchell, "Writing Down Every Morsel Doubles Weight Loss," MSNBC.com, July 8, 2008. http://www.msnbc.msn.com/id/25573436/ns/health-diet_and_nutrition/t/writing-down-every-morsel-doubles-weight-loss/.

Chapter 10: Heart Care and Healthy Body Mass Index (BMI)
1. *Reverso,* 2008, s.v. "heart," http://dictionary.reverso.net/english-definition/heart.
2. Dulce Zamora, "Fitness 101: The Absolute Beginner's Guide to Exercise: How to Get Started with an Exercise Program," *MedMD,* February 12, 2008. http://www.webmd.com/fitness-exercise/guide/fitness-beginners-guide (accessed May 2011).
3. Ibid.
4. *First Place 4 Health Member's Guide* (Ventura, CA: Regal Books, 2008), p. 193.
5. American Council on Exercise, "Ready to Run," 2011. http://www.acefitness.org/fitfacts/fitfacts_display.aspx?itemid=2580 (accessed April 2011).
6. Ibid.
7. *First Place 4 Health Member's Guide,* p. 188.

Chapter 11: Strength Training

1. Centers for Disease Control and Prevention, Injury Prevention and Control: Home and Recreational Safety, "Falls Among Older Adults: An Overview," December 8, 2010. http://www.cdc.gov/HomeandRecreationalSafety/Falls/adultfalls.html (accessed April 2011).
2. Ibid.
3. J. A. Stevens, Fatalities and Injuries from Falls Among Older Adults—United States, 1993-2003 and 2001-2005, MMWR 2006a; 55(45), quoted in Centers for Disease Control and Prevention, Injury Prevention and Control: Home and Recreational Safety, "Falls Among Older Adults: An Overview."
4. Centers for Disease Control and Prevention, Injury Prevention and Control: Home and Recreational Safety, "Falls Among Older Adults: An Overview."
5. *First Place 4 Health Member's Guide* (Ventura, CA: Regal Books, 2008), pp. 201-202.
6. Center for Disease Control and Prevention, Injury Prevention and Control: Home and Recreational Safety, "Why Strength Training," February 24, 2011. http://www.cdc.gov/ physicalactivity/growingstronger/why/index.html (accessed March 2011).
7. *First Place 4 Health Member's Guide*, p. 202.
8. Ibid.
9. Ibid.
10. Ibid., pp. 202-203.
11. Ibid., p. 203.

Chapter 12: Flexibility and Stretching

1. *First Place 4 Health Member's Guide* (Ventura, CA: Regal Books, 2008), p. 206.
2. Ibid., p. 205.
3. Ibid.
4. Oswald Chambers, *My Utmost for His Highest* (Grand Rapids, MI: Discovery House Publishing, 1992), May 8.

Don't Quit—
Get Motivated to
Wellness Today!

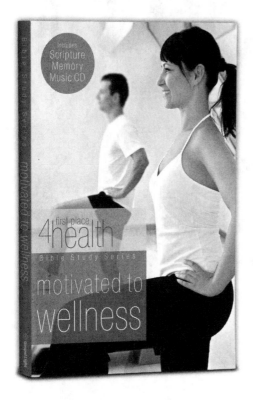

Good health doesn't start with healthy eating and regular exercise. The balanced life so many people long for—which inlcudes good nutrition and physical fitness—begins with a change of heart and a transformed mind. *Motivated to Wellness*, a First Place 4 Health **companion Bible Study to** *Don't Quit, Get Fit*, will invite you to discover hope and motivation that will sustain you through a lifetime of fitness and good health.

motivated to wellness contains:

- Ten weeks of targeted Bible study designed to guide you toward balance and wholeness in every area of life
- Two weeks of menus with grocery lists, original recipes and nutritional information
- Live It Trackers, to document your fitness and eating patterns
- Scripture memory cards
- Scripture memory music CD
- Group prayer request forms
- Prayer partner forms
- Personal weight and measurement record

Motivated to Wellness
ISBN 978.08307.61340

The companion Bible Study to
Don't Quit, Get Fit

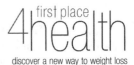

Gospel Light
The Bible. Pure and Simple.
www.gospellight.com

Available at Bookstores Everywhere!
Learn more about the First Place 4 Health program and products at www.firstplace4health.com.

first place
4health
discover a new way to weight loss

First Place 4 Health
Member's Kit

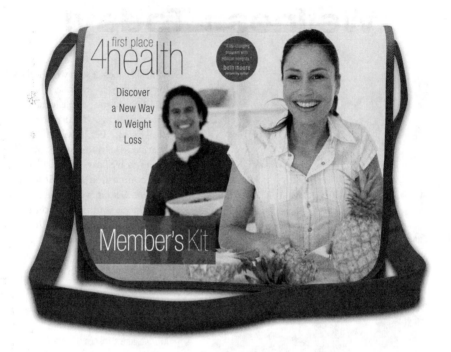

The *First Place 4 Health Member's Kit* contains everything you need to live healthy, lose weight and experience spiritual growth. With each resource, you will learn how to make positive changes in your thoughts and emotions while transforming the way you fuel and recharge your bodies and relate to God.

The Member's Kit includes the following:

- *First Place 4 Health Member's Guide*
- First Place 4 Health (hardcover book)
- *Simple Ideas for Healthy Living*
- *Food-on-the-Go Pocket Guide*
- *Why Should Christians Be Physically Fit?* DVD

- *Emotions & Eating* DVD
- *First Place 4 Health Prayer Journal*
- Member Navigation Sheet

Only $99.99 (a $120 value!)
ISBN 978.08307.60565

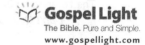

Gospel Light
The Bible. Pure and Simple.
www.gospellight.com

Available at Bookstores Everywhere!
Learn more about the First Place 4 Health program
and products at www.firstplace4health.com.

4 first place
health
discover a new way to weight loss

First Place 4 Health
Group Starter Kit

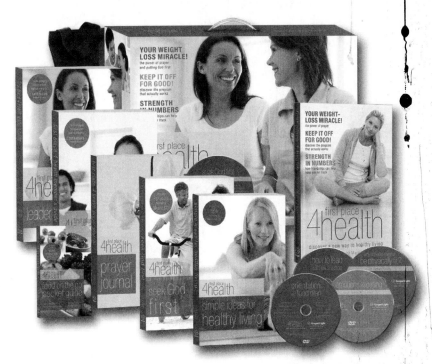

The *First Place 4 Health Group Starter Kit* includes everything you need to confidently lead your group into healthy living, weight loss and spiritual growth. You will find lesson plans, training DVDs, a user-friendly food plan and other easy-to-use tools to help you lead members into a new way of thinking about health.

The Group Starter Kit includes the following:

- A complete *First Place 4 Health Member's Kit*
- *First Place 4 Health Leader's Guide*
- *Seek God First* Bible Study
- *First Place 4 Health Orientation and Food Plan* DVD
- *How to Lead with Excellence* DVD

Only $199.99 (a $256 value!)
ISBN 978.08307.45906

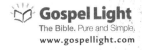

Gospel Light
The Bible. Pure and Simple.
www.gospellight.com

Available at Bookstores Everywhere!
Learn more about the First Place 4 Health program and products at www.firstplace4health.com.

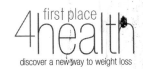

discover a new way to weight loss